Caring

— for Your —

Aging
Parents

Caring
— *for Your* —
Aging
Parents

A Planning and Action Guide

Formerly titled *Seven Steps to Effective Parent Care*

Donna Cohen, Ph.D., and
Carl Eisdorfer, Ph.D., M.D.

A Jeremy P. Tarcher/Putnam Book
published by
G. P. Putnam's Sons
New York

For Bertha and Joe, Dorothy and Sam,
whose legacy of love still lives in the family
D.C.

For Jill and those caring friends
who helped Marc complete his being
C.E.

Permissions and citations appear on pages v–vi.

A Jeremy P. Tarcher / Putnam Book
Published by G. P. Putnam's Sons
Publishers Since 1838
200 Madison Avenue
New York, NY 10016
http://www.putnam.com/putnam

First trade paperback edition 1995

Copyright © 1993 by Professor Donna Cohen, Ph.D., and Carl Eisdorfer, Ph.D., M.D.

Published simultaneously in Canada

Library of Congress Cataloging-in-Publication Data

Cohen, Donna.
    Caring for your aging parents: a planning and action guide / Donna Cohen and Carl Eisdorfer.
        p.   cm.
    "A Jeremy P. Tarcher/Putnam book."
    Includes bibliographical references and index.
    ISBN 0-87477-799-2
    1. Aging parents—Care—United States. 2. Parent and adult child—United States. I. Eisdorfer, Carl. II. Title.
HQ1064.U5C519   1993   93-16267 CIP
306.874—dc20

Design by Lee Fukui

Cover design by Tanya Maiboroda

Printed in the United States of America
    4   5   6   7   8   9   10

This book is printed on acid-free paper.

PERMISSIONS AND CITATIONS

The authors gratefully acknowledge their colleagues, other scholars, and publishers for making possible the inclusion in this work of invaluable information and materials as referenced below:

p. 31: Angel, Marc D., *The Orphaned Adult*, Insight Books: New York, 1987; p. 40: Reiss, David. "The Working Family: A Researcher's View of Health in the Household," *American Journal of Psychology*, 1982, 139; 1412–1420; p. 50: Horowitz, M. J., "Psychological Response to Serious Life Events," from *Human Stress and Cognition: An Information Processing Approach*. V. Hamilton and D. M. Werburton, editors, Wiley: New York, 1979, 235–263; p. 82: Boszormenyi-Nagy, Ivan and Spark, Geraldine M., *Invisible Loyalties: Reciprocity in Intergenerational Family Therapy*, Harper & Row, Hagerstown, Maryland, 1973 (RC 488.5 B65 1973 FMHI); p. 94: Radloff, Lenora S., "The CES-D Scale: A Self-Report Depression Scale for Research in the General Population," from *Applied Psychological Measurement*, 1977; pp. 95–97: The American Cancer Society, *Tips for Coping With Depression*, pamphlet; pp. 101–102: Beck, Aaron T., M.D., and Emery, Gary, Ph.D., *Anxiety Disorders and Phobias*, Copyright 1985 by Aaron T. Beck, M.D. and Gary Emery, Ph.D. Reprinted by permission of Basic Books, a division of HarperCollins Publishers, Inc.; p. 103: Ryan, Regina Sara, *The Fine Art of Recuperation*, Jeremy P. Tarcher, Inc., Los Angeles, 1989; pp. 115–117: Haly, William E., Clair, Jeffrey M., and Soulsberg, Karen, "Family Caregiver Satisfaction With Medical Care of Their Demented Relatives," from *The Gerontologist*, 1992, 32: 219–226; pp. 118–119: Harris H. McIlwain, Cori F. Steinmeyer, Debra Fulghum Bruce, R. E. Fulghum, and Robert G. Bruce, *The 50+ Wellness Program*, 1990 John Wiley & Sons. Reprinted by permission of John Wiley & Sons, Inc.; pp. 159–161: George, Linda, *The Duke University Caregiver Well-Being Survey*, Duke University, 1987. With permission of Linda George; pp. 162–163: The Wien Center, a joint program of The Mount Sinai Medical Center and The University of Miami School of Medicine, *Self-Esteem Assessment*. With permission of The Mount Sinai Medical Center, Florida; pp. 165–168: Adapted from *Stress & Health*, 2nd Edition, by Philip L. Rice. Copyright 1992, 1987 by Wadsworth, Inc. Adapted by permission of Brooks/Cole Publishing Company, Pacific Grove, CA 93950; pp. 168–169: Mefall, Stephanie and Miller, Baila H., "Caregiver Burden and Nursing Home Admission of Frail Elderly Persons," from *The Journal of Gerontology, Social Sciences*, 1992, 47: 573–579. Adapted from the National Long Term Care Survey of 1982 which is in the Public Domain. With permission of Ms. Mefall; pp. 172–174: Holines, Thomas and Rahe, Richard H., "The Social Readjustment Scale," from *The Journal of Psychometric Research*, 1967, 11: 213–218. Reprinted with permission from Pergamon Press Ltd., Oxford, England; pp. 186–187: Nancy Neveloff Dubler and David Nimmons, *Ethics on Call: A Medical Ethicist Shows How to Take Charge of Life-and-Death Choices*. Copyright 1992 by Nancy Neveloff Dubler and David Nimmons. Reprinted by permission of Harmony Books, a division of Crown Publishers, Inc.; pp. 190–191: Morycyz, Richard, *Research on Aging*, 7:3, 1985, 329–361. Copyright 1985. Reprinted by permission of Sage Publications, Inc.; pp. 191–202: Nancy Neveloff Dubler and David Nimmons, *Ethics on Call: A Medical Ethicist Shows How to Take Charge of Life-and-Death Choices*. Copyright 1992 by Nancy Neveloff Dubler and David Nimmons. Reprinted by permission of Harmony Books, a division of Crown Publishers, Inc.; pp. 202–203: Harris H. McIlwain, Cori F. Steinmeyer, Debra Fulghum Bruce, R. E. Fulghum, and Robert G. Bruce. *The 50+ Wellness Program*, 1990 John Wiley & Sons. Reprinted by permission of John Wiley & Sons, Inc.

ACKNOWLEDGMENTS

Acknowledgments are often the last and most difficult part to compose in a book. Many different people and circumstances shaped the writing of this book, and it is impossible to list everyone. We are especially indebted to the thousands of older persons and their families whose identities must be disguised but whose lives have touched us deeply. There are no words to express adequately our appreciation to them. We are grateful to Jeremy Tarcher, who was so passionate about the importance of publishing this book. Rick Benzel was a provocative editor whose energy and arguments helped shape the text. As a result this book has a special quality reflecting Rick's blood and sweat, as well as our own.

Our own families gave us a very precious gift—the time to work together. Our many friends and colleagues read parts of the manuscript and made very helpful suggestions. Two dear friends, both of whom died too young, inspired us with their ideas, their courage, and their own ability to care for others during sickness and death: Stuart Golan and Jean Cahn, we miss you.

Three people typed and retyped the manuscript with tender loving care—Nan O'Hanlon, Joyce Johnson, and Judy Toole. They were fiercely possessive of its growth and development, as was Adrienne Jaret, and their tears and laughter shaped our editing. Finally, we appreciate Judy Perry, who devoted hours to reading and rereading the text.

This book was especially difficult to finish in the summer of

1992. Marc Adam Eisdorfer died on July 4, after four years with AIDS. Marc, you are remembered every day by your father, the rest of your family, and friends. Your life and death showed us that caring is more than loving. May you rest in peace.

CONTENTS

PREFACE

This book will help you to meet the challenges of caring for your aging parents. A wide variety of self-help books and manuals for adult children who are caring for aging parents are readily available. This book is different. It describes a new way of thinking about your role in caring and does not duplicate much of what is found in other books. Our focus is on your need to address the challenges you face, to organize and balance your life, and to help others collaborate with you in caring.

Caring for Your Aging Parents, as its title suggests, maps a route to effective caregiving, with guidelines for planning and implementing your caregiving activities and solving many of your problems. We alert you to the issues that you must examine before help can be brought in. When your older parents become frail, sick, or disabled, your life changes. New commitments emerge whether you love them, dislike them, or are indifferent to them. Whatever your feelings and circumstances, you are faced with a fundamental problem—how to do the right thing while balancing your obligations to everyone else, including yourself, in the way that works best for your family.

Parent-caring has become a normal part of family life. On any given day it is estimated that as many as 10 million Americans are engaged in "carefrontations," or situations of stress and strain that adult children and other family members experience while caring for aging parents. It is a rare household where all family members manage to agree on what is right all the time without arguments.

As many as nine out of ten adult children report having major conflicts with other family members around the care of an older parent.

Families change and reorganize as people are born, grow old, and die. As we live longer and spend more time together, however, these extended interdependencies—between parents and children, brothers and sisters, husbands and wives, parents and grandparents, and grandparents and grandchildren—create new obligations and commitments. With more older persons requiring help, more adult children are paying the emotional as well as the financial bills of our changing family patterns.

Our society has not yet evolved strategies to help the rapidly increasing number of adult children who are responsible for the care of the older generation while at the same time caring for themselves and the younger generation. In the United States parents are legally responsible for their children, but obligations for parent-caring are rarely mandated. Adult children's responsibilities to their parents are based on ethical and moral claims that vary from family to family and from culture to culture. Yet it is well recognized that these responsibilities affect the morale, productivity, health, and absenteeism of many workers across the country. Lacking preparation and clear guidelines for what is appropriate, many caregivers are left full of anger, shame, and guilt as they wrestle with how much they can and should do for their older parents.

We have been working with older persons and their family members for decades, and we have been doing so together since 1976. For this book we have used the results of our family research projects and clinical programs at Duke University in Durham, North Carolina, the University of Washington in Seattle, the Albert Einstein College of Medicine and the Montefiore Medical Center in New York, the University of Miami, and the University of Illinois at Chicago.

We thus bring a broad perspective on aging to this book, based on our extensive research and clinical experience. At Duke University, Carl was a pioneer in identifying the emerging impact of aging on our society. His work on the normal intellectual changes of advancing age and on Alzheimer's disease helped identify the growing issues that individuals and families face as the older population grows in number and proportion of society. Donna became interested in aging as a student of Carl's at Duke. She developed her own studies of the biobehavioral aspects of cognitive changes with aging and Alzheimer's disease at the University of Southern California and at the University of California at Los Angeles. We began our now-longstanding collaboration when Donna joined the faculty of the department of psychiatry and behavioral sciences at the University of Washington in 1976.

As chairman of the department at the University of Washington, Carl established a number of programs for older persons and their families. The outpatient Geriatric Family Service and the inpatient unit at the American Lake Veterans Hospital for persons with Alzheimer's disease and related disorders have become models for clinical care throughout the country. Working with family members coming to these programs, we began to understand the many pressures that result from caring for aging relatives with mental and physical problems. We were also instrumental in the development of ASIST—the Alzheimer Support and Information Service Team—one of seven family support groups in the United States that together gave birth to the National Alzheimer's Disease and Related Disorders Association, now based in Chicago.

We continued our collaboration in New York from 1981 through 1985. As head of the Division of Aging and Geriatric Psychiatry at the Albert Einstein College of Medicine and the Montefiore Medical Center, Donna not only replicated several of the clinical programs from Seattle, including the original Geriatric Family Service, but greatly expanded the family treatment and support components. One of the most important findings from our clinical research during this period was that depression is present in more than half of primary caregivers of relatives with Alzheimer's disease. Many investigators have since replicated these findings. It is now well documented that caring for older relatives—not just those with Alzheimer's disease—is stressful and can have a negative impact on the mental and physical health of caregivers.

Continuing our research and clinical activities, Donna in

Chicago and Carl in Miami, we focused on ways to help family members cope with aging relatives as well as to empower older people to participate in their own care. Funded by a grant from the National Institute on Aging, under Donna's leadership and involving clinical researchers at six other medical centers, we interviewed family caregivers to study the factors that predicted who would succumb to the stress of caregiving and who would stay healthy. This research increased our understanding of the risks associated with caring, and we wrote this book to help families learn to deal effectively with the problems of caregiving, reduce their emotional distress, and remain healthy and productive.

Perhaps the most important thing we learned is that caring is not the same as loving. Many of us think that caring is easy as long as we love the person we are caring for, but it is not. Caring involves specific skills—looking and listening, planning, showing empathy, thinking through problems, taking appropriate actions, and working with others. We are not born with these skills; nor do we develop them naturally out of love. They must be learned, be it at home, in a hospital or nursing home, at school, or at the workplace. Caring takes different forms, and there are different needs in caring relationships between different people—infants and adults, marriage partners, friends, and between children and aged parents.

How should you care for your aging parents and other relatives? There is no absolute answer. What you will do depends on your parents' needs and on you, your family, and your circumstances. Therefore, what we offer here is a framework to learn how to care more effectively. We describe ways to look and listen as well as think and act when aging parents need help. At times we will discuss issues as if they were simple. We know that family life is never simple, however, and that decisions do not always result in everyone's happiness. The simplicity of some of our discussions is intended to illustrate the specific steps everyone can take, even in the most painful and demanding situations.

Being prepared for problems—having a plan and knowing what to do—not only leads to effective caregiving but can prevent the overwhelming sense of hopelessness and helplessness that affects so many caregivers. Experiencing hopelessness and isolation in dealing with longstanding pressures leads some family members, tragically, to take their own life and that of their loved one. Although accurate data are not available, a number of well-publicized murder-suicides or double suicides involving older couples have brought public attention to the extreme depression that often accompanies caring for someone you love.

Throughout the book we have related many stories to illustrate how other people have taken control and done something. These stories are intended to show that there are different ways to succeed and that success is relative. Whatever you and your family do may not meet your expectations or those of your parents and others around you. If it is the best you can do in your cirumstances, however, this book can help you learn to accept these limitations and feel some satisfaction or peace of mind that you have tried your best.

The stories in this book are not about any single person or family. In order to maintain confidentiality, to protect and respect the privacy of those who have shared their lives with us, we have synthesized and merged details from many families, including letters, conversations, and diary entries. The stories do not suggest there are any right or wrong answers. What worked for one family may not work for yours.

We make specific suggestions for dealing with complex and sometimes painful circumstances, but every family is a fabric of invisible bonds and often-unrecognized family loyalties and tensions leading to conflict, indifference, estrangement, and violence as well as to love, joy, and mutual commitment. Our stories portray the complexity of family crises from many perspectives, and by doing this, we emphasize that everyone in a family is affected and that everyone must come to grips with an older relative's illness, decline, or death in their own way.

We hope this book will help address the emerging public concern about long-term care and the shared responsibilities among families and communities for those who are dependent and chronically ill. The perversity of our current fragmented system of health care and the lack of access to appropriate and affordable human services are a strain for most of us. This is particularly true in the United States, but it is also a problem in many other countries. As the world population ages rapidly and people depend on one another longer, the burden of health and human services will not only challenge the resources of many countries but potentially undermine the strength and health of families everywhere. We must recognize that our actions today will affect not only the quality of our lives but the quality of our children's and our grandchildren's lives.

Another message of this book may best be understood by those who have already gone through the experience of caring for an aging parent. It is often painful to face change as we grow older, and it is not easy to alter our lives to accommodate others, especially when their dependency and disability have lasted for many years or when family relationships have been estranged or indifferent for some time. If we can deal with the pain of those challenges, however, as well as with the often-insoluble dilemmas presented to us by increasing longevity, we can achieve the extraordinary reward of being human—to learn and grow wiser as we ourselves grow older.

Overview: Seven Steps to Effective Caregiving

The traditional view of parent-caring needs overhauling. Adult children are not and can never be parents to their own aging parents. You are not mothering Mom or fathering Dad. Whatever your parents' problems, they are not children. They are adult members of your family who have specific needs as they grow old, and you are an adult child who is also growing older. You have personal needs as well as responsibilities for other people in your life as well as for your parents. In order to respond to parents who are frail, sick, or disabled, you have a series of choices to make about their care. You must make decisions about whether you will get involved, how much, for how long, at what cost, and to what end. Caring requires you to take actions that are often ambiguous, painful, and confusing. And confusion is a barrier to action.

This book presents a seven-step framework for learning how to be effective when aging parents need care. The seven steps are not part of a recipe for instant success, but they are components of an overall strategy to achieve what we call caregiver "effectivity." Your effectivity is your ability to figure out the right thing to do for your parents, to manage your resources to do what needs to be done, and to be flexible and change your course when necessary. Therefore, effectivity is a continuing process of enhancing effectiveness. The seven steps segment the process in order to achieve effectivity so that you can lay out your course one step at a time.

The first step is to recognize the problems that exist and prioritize them. This sounds simple, but it is not. Every aspect of your personal and family life may be affected by your caregiving, and you may feel overwhelmed by what seems to be insurmountable problems. You may ignore or overlook problems and rely on familiar ways to reduce your immediate distress. Learning to recognize difficulties and sort out your priorities will allow you to begin to organize yourself for the task ahead of you.

The second step is to overcome your feelings of denial. Denial may take many forms. It can involve minimizing or avoiding a problem, or refusing to recognize that you can make a difference. People commonly deny something is happening when it is serious or harmful. Denial protects you and gives you the time to recover from a shock or a painful experience. In most cases, however, denial must be eventually worked through so that legitimate emotions of anger, sadness, confusion, and anxiety can be dealt with and resolved.

Overcoming denial is the basis for moving successfully to the third step—managing your emotions. Emotions are a wonderful part of being human, and everyone experiences a range of feelings, from pleasure and happiness to sadness, fear, and anger. Persistent and uncontrolled depression, anxiety, and anger will not only make you miserable but will interfere with successful caregiving as well.

The fourth step is building collaborations or partnerships. Your partners may include other family members, health care professionals, workers from community agencies, lawyers, financial advisers, and others. An important element in building partnerships is to know your assets and to identify what kinds of help you will need. Locating the right people and services means finding reliable sources of information and referral. Once you have found these resources, you may need to develop the skills to develop collaborative relationships with those able to provide help.

The fifth step is learning to balance the competing needs of your parents and others who are dependent on you. This is an ongoing process, and it may become more and more difficult as time goes on. As parents become more needy, it becomes necessary to reallocate family resources equitably, including time and money.

The sixth step is learning crisis skills to help when you feel out of control. Crises will always occur during the course of caregiving, and amidst the turmoil you will have opportunities for growth and new learning if you can learn how to regain control, including getting outside help.

The final and seventh step is letting go, moving on with your life, and learning to accept that you have done your best. This process occurs differently for every person and in every family. As older parents deteriorate and die, letting go is especially painful and difficult when they are suffering and death is prolonged. Letting go is a complicated process that also means finding ways to distance yourself from the situation, finding time for yourself and pleasurable pursuits, as well as letting others help you. After parents have died, there are specific strategies you can follow to come to terms with what you could or could not do, as well as to get on with the rest of your life.

Caring is a way of thinking and acting interdependently with the people of your life. Love is a potent force, but love does not always lead to effective caring. It is not necessary to love your parents to care for them, but it is essential to deal with them effectively in some way. Meeting the endless needs of someone you love deeply may become impossible as illness and death take their course and evoke painful feelings. On the other hand, having to address the needs of someone you do not love leads to problems. When caring is thought of as the responsibility for acting effectively over time—with "effectivity"—it becomes an attainable goal. Using the seven steps to increase your effectivity as a caregiver will take time and practice, but you can develop these skills to make and implement better decisions with and for your aging parents and other family members.

COMMON CAREGIVING DILEMMAS

Over the past fifteen years we have been impressed by how much adult children do for their aging parents when adversity threatens mobility, health, security, comfort, and overall well-being. There are many problems to be solved—complex and often painful problems. Many family members master these problems, but sadly we have seen just as many who, despite well-intentioned efforts, fail.

Family members have described a variety of difficult problems. Perhaps these examples sound familiar:

My mother is getting too sick to take care of Dad anymore. She refuses to put him in a nursing home. She won't move in with us, and she refuses outside help.

The neighborhood my parents live in has changed. It's not safe anymore. Dad has been mugged once, and the house was broken into last month. However, both Mom and Dad refuse to move.

Dad can't live alone anymore. Ever since his stroke he has needed a lot of assistance. My brother has been paying for home care but doesn't want to keep footing the bill. He wants me to help out, but I don't want to. I don't like my father. He was a mean and hurtful person all his life.

Mom has been dependent on me for over twenty years, ever since Dad died. Her health is getting worse, and she is becoming more demanding. It's impossible to please her, even though I visit every day and do a thousand and one things for her. In fact, everyone in the family is trying to help her. Yet she still tells everyone who will listen that the family has deserted her.

Mom's cancer is spreading rapidly, and the prognosis is bleak. She had a pulmonary crisis, and they transferred her to the ICU. I know she doesn't want to go on like this. She asked us to let her die at home with no extraordinary rescues.

I may have to quit my job to spend time with Dad. He has Alzheimer's disease and needs a lot of help, but we need my salary to cover family expenses.

Mom is dead now, and all of us feel guilty for putting her in a nursing home. Every time we saw her, she was depressed and crying. We should have done more for her.

Although there are no easy prescriptions for solving these dilemmas and many others, this book describes a method of organizing your situation to deal with the difficult tasks involved. There is nothing magical about the seven steps, but they are a simple and useful way to compartmentalize the complexities of caregiving into manageable parts in order to find solutions to problems.

This simple approach is needed because so many people will be living longer in our society, and we know little about what this will mean. The phenomenon of growing old together across many generations is as widespread as it is new and is leading our society into new frontiers in human relationships. Increasing longevity creates more time for family members to know and be involved with one another, but it also creates the opportunity for more things to go wrong, as well as opportunities for a reversal of the usual pattern of caring, from parent to child to child to parent.

This book can be thought of as a personal survival manual. It takes courage to change and learn new things about yourself and your family to make difficult decisions when your aging parents need help. It can be scary, painful, costly, and burdensome, but we also believe that it can be a rewarding experience.

An Example of the Opportunities of Caregiving

We will try to introduce you to the potential for new learning and change in caregiving through excerpts from a series of letters written by Sharon Baker, a forty-five-year-old woman, to her younger sister, Debbie. Over the years Sharon wrote Debbie many letters that together describe the odyssey of a woman juggling responsibilities for her mother and father, her husband, her children, and herself.

Dear Sis,

I am writing you now because my spirit is too sore to speak. Dad is wasting away day by day and Mom is getting too frail to care for him.

Dad should go into a nursing home, but Mom refuses. She is too crippled to care for him alone, and we can't continue to pay for round-the-clock care after December. This is not a request for money—we know the situation at your place. I just needed to share my feelings with you.

Jack and I want her to live with us and place Dad in a nursing home close by. Mom insists they can't leave their friends, and since they live more than a thousand miles away, I feel helpless. I can't allow them to go on as they are, yet I cannot afford to fly there every weekend.

I want to do what is right and best for them . . . but I'm not sure what to do.

Sharon wrote these lines several weeks before she and her husband, Jack, made the decision to move her parents into their own home. Sharon confessed that the decision seemed obvious once it was made: "I realized I had to do what my heart told me to do. I could have let the situation get worse, or I could have brought my parents close where we could do something to help them. I had to learn to tell my mother how I felt and what I was thinking. I also had to ask her to tell me what she was feeling and thinking. In order to discover the way to change her world and mine, we had to go through a difficult process—something I can only call mutual education. It was awkward and harrowing at times because as daughter and mother we had to break down old barriers and learn about each other as different people, as a daughter and mother who had grown older."

Many of Sharon's early letters, written before she decided to bring her parents to her home, contained outpourings of defused anger, profound grief, and a sense of hopelessness and inadequacy at being caught in the middle.

Dear Deb,

I know what it feels like to go crazy. Night after night now I have cried into my pillow. I feel stuck in a web of people, places, and emotions.

Mom and Dad need me, but Jack is adamant that I stop flying there every weekend. We had an awful fight last week, and I was almost ready to move out of the house because he was being so unreasonable.

I am angry with him, my parents . . . and I am even angry with the dog for needing me to feed him every night. I'm trying to do everything for everyone, but it's not working. I've lost my sense of balance.

Caring is emotional business, and unless you can learn to recognize and manage your emotions, it will be difficult for you to deal with your problems. This is true of challenges across the life span—sustaining a marriage, raising children, working productively, developing friendships, and helping family members and friends. Quite often there are many surprises, and some of them can teach us to see ourselves and our loved ones in different ways.

Several months after Sharon's parents moved into their home, her father had another stroke. At this point Sharon decided to leave her job and do freelance writing at home. Their hours together provided her with opportunities to learn about the man who was her father:

Dear Deb,

I know I am living by a clock that has no hands. I want to go back to work, but Dad has so little time left. My life will only go forward again if I can say good-bye to him "the right way." He needs me now to care for him the way he has always protected everyone else.

Dad has begun to talk about life in Russia—how he and his brothers and sisters survived the riots, enduring until they could endure no more. In these precious hours I am seeing our father as another person. When we were young, Dad worked long hours, and then we grew up, married, and raised our own families.

These last months have been a gift of time, the time to learn about each other.

After her father died, Sharon went back to work, and her mother continued to live with them. Sharon's letters to Debbie related how daughter and mother were learning to understand each other. These letters were not without their sadness and frustration, and they described the paralyzing inertia of inaction. They also chronicled the process of how an adult child and her mother could transcend the burden of past relationships and the painful assaults of chronic illness to reconnect with each other:

> Dear Deb,
>
> I never thought Mom appreciated me and what I was doing with my life. Last week when we rushed her to the hospital, I realized for the first time that she might die. And I think Mom sensed the same thing.
>
> I have spent every day at the hospital, and Mom and I have begun to talk in ways that I never thought possible. Last night Mom told me how ashamed she was of being sick and unable to do things for herself. She also reached out to hug me. She said I made her feel loved and wanted even though she was wasting away.
>
> Then Mom asked me to forgive her for not being a good mother. Deb, I suddenly realized that I did love her. Thank God I found out in time!

Caring for your aging parents will teach you new things about yourself and your parents, even if your relationship with them has been distant or hostile in the past. Despite the courage this requires, the rewards can be incalculable. People like Sharon can teach us to be optimistic about a future where more and more people will be living longer. Family members who are successful in coping with the needs of their aging parents recognize that they cannot resolve problems except by *trying* to solve them!

SEVEN STEPS TO EFFECTIVE CAREGIVING

Caring for aging parents usually means coping with changes for a long time. The seven steps listed below provide a framework to cope effectively with these successive changes over time:

Step 1.   Recognize and prioritize problems

Step 2.   Overcome denial

Step 3.   Manage emotions

Step 4.   Build collaborative partnerships

Step 5. Balance needs and resources

Step 6. Take control in a crisis

Step 7. Let go and move on

These steps are intended to help you anticipate and examine the scope of work ahead of you and make it manageable. Sometimes the magnitude of parent-caring problems feels overwhelming because the problems will continue for your parents' lifetime and are added to your own problems.

The following story about Cathy Jordan and her family illustrates the seven steps before we describe them in depth in the ensuing chapters. Cathy had been wrestling with her parents' health problems and her concern that they had not been taking care of themselves for more than a decade. We introduce her situation and the complexities of caregiving with part of a letter written to a younger sister, Ann, who lived abroad:

Dear Ann,

My memories of our childhood are wonderful . . . Dad out in the corn fields, Mom brushing your hair on the porch, Bob and me chasing each other in the yard, Ginger cradling her pet chicken, and the wind blowing ever so gently.

But that world is gone now. The farm is run down, and weeds have overrun our old vegetable garden. Mom and Dad are not what they used to be. Day after day, they stay in the house and cook and eat like there is no tomorrow.

Mom's diabetes has been out of control since the cancer operation. She has lost sight in both of her eyes and doesn't care about living anymore. I tried to tell Dad that if Mom doesn't watch her diet, she may have another stroke or go into a coma.

If it happens to Mom, we will have another problem . . . finding a place for Ginger. I can't believe she was fifty-two years old last week, and harder to believe, Dad still blames Mom's diabetes for her being retarded.

What are we going to do? I can't keep her! And I know you're in no position, either. I don't know what to do, but I keep hoping that everything will work out.

Cathy had become increasingly frustrated with her family problems—her parents' chronic illnesses and destructive health behaviors, the future of her developmentally disabled sister, and the needs of her own children. As the oldest daughter and the one who lived closest to her parents, Cathy had tried many times and in many ways to get her parents to take better care of themselves, but with no success. Ann lived abroad, and the letters Cathy wrote her were an important outlet for her frustration. Cathy's husband, John, was supportive, but she was determined not to burden him too much. John Jordan worked two jobs to support the family as it was. She thought it was her "job" to take care of family matters.

Cathy tried to resign herself to what was happening. Her parents were both in their early seventies, they had been married for more than fifty years, and they were responsible for their own lives even though they were hurting themselves. Cathy, a strong-willed individual, usually did everything she set out to accomplish, but it was breaking her heart that she was powerless when it came to her parents. As time passed, she not only became increasingly angry with them, she blamed herself for being inadequate.

Cathy's mother finally had a serious stroke. To everyone's surprise, she survived—but with paralysis, speech problems, and considerable cognitive impairment. After a long hospitalization, the doctors recommended that the family consider placing her in a nursing home. Cathy was fortunate to find a nursing home that took Medicaid patients and that was also close enough for her father to visit. Cathy wrote to Ann and described her sense of satisfaction that she had finally been able to accomplish something:

> Strange as it sounds, it's a relief to get Mom into a home. Even Dad has accepted the arrangement, although he threatened to disown me for doing this to her and him.

Cathy Jordan's story illustrates many common circumstances that adult caregivers face. Such responsibilities often fall to the oldest daughter or daughter-in-law. Geographic distance impacts the ability of families to share the responsibilities. Caregiving can go on for a very long period of time. It can also be extremely difficult, if not impossible, to convince parents to adopt health-promoting behaviors, especially when very old and sick parents have given up the desire to live and care for themselves. Developmentally disabled older persons who have grown old living with their parents are not rare, and their future well-being is threatened when their aging parents are less able to care for them. Finally, finding a good nursing home can be tough, especially when parents and others blame you for not caring enough, but nursing homes are legitimate options among others in the spectrum of long-term care services.

Although Cathy eventually became consumed by attending to the many needs of her parents, she had known her parents were aging for several years, but despite a long history of various problems, she had never felt the responsibility to step into her parents' life before. Recognizing the problem is the first step to effective caring.

Step 1: Recognize and Prioritize Problems

The first step is to recognize that you have problems and what they are. This seems simple, as we have said, but it is almost always a complex issue. At the risk of oversimplification, problems occur in two time frames—acute and insidious. An acute time frame involves a sudden emergency call after an accident, fall, or stroke, and there is little doubt about the person's immediate need for help. Whose help is needed may be a source of conflict or confusion, but the fact that help is suddenly needed creates an acute problem. Interventions are immediate, and the question of whether to intervene gives way to the question of how to best provide the necessary assistance.

Aging is a gradual process, however, and many infirmities of later life appear slowly. The memory lapses and unusual behaviors that often characterize Alzheimer's disease and related brain disorders take place in an insidious time frame. The progression of arthritis with decreased mobility and painful joints slowly incapacitates once active and vibrant bodies. The loss of purchasing power while living with a fixed income in an inflationary economy, in a changing neighborhood, and with increasing frailty have an enormous impact on an older person's life, but these changes may be imperceptible from day to day or even from month to month.

There are many challenges in recognizing a problem with an insidious onset. One of the greatest is that aging parents may deny the need for assistance, even when their condition is serious. Many parents do not want to be a burden, insisting that they can function independently. Many feel that their problems are normal and are simply the result of "old age." Perhaps one of the greatest difficulties that adult children have is feeling that they need to do something when their parents do not agree that a problem exists.

Complicating these issues is the likelihood that you are facing not just one but many problems, as Cathy Jordan was, especially as your parents deteriorate. Therefore, this first step sets the stage for a continuing process of monitoring change over time.

STEP 2. OVERCOME DENIAL

When problems arise, family members often minimize a parent's unusual behavior, complaints, or increasing demands, as "par for the course" or part of "normal aging." It is not unusual to deny that anything is really wrong, even as circumstances change. As Cathy's mother slowly lost her eyesight and developed other complications, for example, Cathy did not believe that diabetes was the issue for a time. Rather, she focused on her mother's age, believing that people generally lose their vision and get sick as they grow old.

Cathy's beliefs are not unusual. People often work very hard to manage the needs of their parents yet still deny the problem. Many refuse to accept for a long time that their parents are headed for trouble. Years before her mother's first stroke, Cathy had thought the farm looked shoddy and that her parents were eating and drinking excessively. But their lives had always revolved around food, and they had always been overweight. Likewise, the farm had been in the family for more than a hundred eighty years, and the house and barn were old! But Cathy could not bring herself to recognize the problem. At some point, however, wishful-beliefs that things are normal cannot be maintained. Usually a critical event occurs that disrupts business-as-usual activities and coping patterns that have worked in the past. Whatever the critical event, it causes a number of feelings to surface, including fear, anger, anxiety, and confusion. Concerned family members ask questions to obtain information and figure out what is wrong, but usually do not know where to turn for assistance.

For Cathy, the critical event was not her mother's first stroke. It was an interaction between her ten-year-old son, Dan, and her mother that occurred on Thanksgiving, several weeks before the stroke. Cathy and Dan were setting the table when her parents began an angry fight in the kitchen. Cathy's mother barged into the dining room and screamed at Cathy that no one loved her and that she wanted to die. At that point Dan moved toward his grandmother and reached for her arm, saying "But I love you, and I won't let you die!" His grandmother slapped his face and shouted, "I wish you were dead too!" It was then that Cathy finally realized that something was drastically wrong with her mother, who had never laid a hand on anybody. She knew it was time to seek help.

Step 3. Manage Emotions

Caring is an emotional business, and learning to recognize when your emotions are clouding your good judgment and perhaps affecting your health is important. In several studies, half or more of all caregivers living with relatives needing substantial care became depressed enough to need clinical help. If this is the case with you, your family, friends, and clergy can help you deal with your feelings. You can also get professional help in overcoming your problems before they get worse. It is common sense to go to a doctor or dentist before a health problem becomes serious. It makes similar good sense to get help before emotional dilemmas get so bad that they interfere with your ability to get things done.

Although Cathy Jordan developed no major depression or other significant health problems, she experienced significant distress and often blamed herself for not being good enough. There were many days when significant conflict erupted in her house, as we will describe later.

STEP 4. BUILD COLLABORATIVE PARTNERSHIPS

When things go wrong and aging parents need help, their physical problem needs to be evaluated and diagnosed professionally. A diagnosis, however, can reflect only part of the problem. A person's ability to function is affected not only by their particular disease but by problems with personal care activities, their lifestyle, and the availability of help at home. Since older persons may have many problems, family members must begin to deal with a whole set of issues that loom ahead of them. During this period you must examine resources, roles, and relationships carefully. In addition to getting the correct diagnosis, you need to develop a sense of what appropriate care you will need to provide. The list of resources that your parents will need may range from shopping and laundry to medical care and companionship.

It was after her mother's first stroke and recovery that Cathy and her family understood that the problems her mother experienced had been the result of uncontrolled diabetes, unstable blood pressure, and consequent circulatory problems in the brain. After her mother recovered, however, Cathy watched as her parents reverted to the old behaviors of eating and drinking, ignoring diets, and forgetting to take insulin injections. It was then all too clear to Cathy what lay ahead.

STEP 5. BALANCE NEEDS AND RESOURCES

This is a strategy of developing the skills to effectively balance your competing obligations and responsibilities. Your goal is to assist your parents while minimizing the disruptions in your own life, your work, and your family's habits. Most adult children are willing to change their schedules at work and at home to do what needs to be done, but this can be difficult to do when parents need help over long periods of time. Continuing changes are stressful, and it is unlikely that everyone's needs can be balanced except for brief periods.

Cathy and her family visited her parents regularly, usually around major holidays. After the first stroke, however, she began visiting several times a month, often without the rest of the family. John had to work most weekends, and the kids were growing up with activities of their own. When her family began to complain about her absence, Cathy admonished them for their selfishness and lack of concern for her parents who needed her.

Cathy finally arranged for a homemaker to visit her parents, as well as a chore worker to do minor repairs. Her parents accepted this reluctantly for a while, but finally they asked to be left alone. They could get by on their own, they said, and did not want strangers in their home. Cathy coaxed John and their older sons to do some work on the farm for several months, but this activity stopped because her father was insistent that the family "leave his farm alone!" He even accused them of trying to take the farm away from him and threatened to cut them out of the will.

Effectively balancing the various factors involved, getting people to agree on a plan, and having to change again and again can be aggravating. Increased anger and frustration are common as things get worse, and when emotions run high, you may pressure other family members in ways that drive them away rather than invite them to help you solve the problem.

Cathy tried every possible avenue to convince her parents they needed to change their lifestyle and accept some help with the farm. She was convinced that her children would have a positive impact on her parents and hopefully cheer them up. This did not happen, however, and the children left to go back home midsummer, upset and angry with their grandparents. Cathy and John argued endlessly and almost separated. She and her sister Ann exchanged angry phone calls as Cathy felt burdened and weary from her battles with everyone and overwhelmed by what she saw as the demands being made on her.

Cathy's way of dealing with her worsening situation was to continue to do the same thing, only more so. Her modus operandi was to demand still more of herself and her family. But increasing these demands had the opposite effect. Her husband and children backed off even more, and the net effect was that she alienated the entire family, including her parents. Instead of making the situation better, her efforts had only made a bad situation worse.

Strategies must change when chronic illness and problems persist. Cathy needed to modify her tactics—to stop, assess what was happening to her parents, husband, and children, and look for another way. In situations like this, when caregivers are persistent in what amounts to destructive interventions, it usually takes a crisis to challenge the family to change, sometimes for the better and sometimes for the worse.

STEP 6. TAKE CONTROL IN A CRISIS

It is common for crises to flare up as the demands of chronic caring take their toll over time. Tensions build, and conflicts disrupt family relationships. Toward the end of the summer, John threatened to leave Cathy if she persisted in spending all of her time with and energy on her parents. Her parents refused to change their ways, and John could not understand why Cathy persisted in beating her head against a wall to provide care that they only rejected. He did not have these problems with his parents.

Cathy and John agreed to stay together for the sake of their children, but a day rarely went by without a disagreement between them. Tensions ran high, and the children developed problems. The youngest child, who had always been a model student, began failing tests and acting out against the teacher and other children. John described what was happening in the family:

> Cathy's parents have been a pain over most of our married life but particularly over the last five years. Getting married and having kids changed our lives, but dealing with her parents has affected us more!
>
> I have always gotten along with them, but it gets harder to have positive thoughts about them because they are so different now. Their health has gotten worse, and they don't seem to care

about anything—themselves, the kids, or us. They have become so unpleasant, there are times when I can't stand being around them. I even cringe when they're on the phone.

As problems persist, family members may eventually find themselves unable to cope. It is not unusual for individuals to turn their attention from the person who is sick to another family member, whom they blame or scapegoat. The family system, no longer able to solve problems or mobilize resources effectively, breaks down. This situation is characterized by angry and often violent behavior as well as by frustration and depression, when caregivers simply cannot stabilize their changing circumstances.

Cathy finally recognized that her own home was falling apart and that her family was in turmoil. Her son Dan was caught during a drug raid on the school grounds. Her middle son, Terry, who was in military school, was placed on probation for cheating on his examinations. Another son, Alan, was fired from his newspaper job for not completing his assignments, and the oldest son, Jason, announced that he was dropping out of college.

John blamed Cathy for the failings of their sons. She had spent so much time with her parents, he said, that she had stopped being a mother to them. Cathy, in turn, was furious with John, accusing him of not being a good father. She herself felt guilty because she had failed with her parents, her children, and her marriage. Cathy became obsessed with her failures: a family that seemed to be falling apart and a future that seemed to be going nowhere. She found herself reacting to what she perceived were her parents' needs, without recognizing the importance of taking control of her life and developing a strategy of care.

Step 7. Let Go and Move On

Letting go occurs in a different way in every family, but certain events occur over time that separate the chronically ill person and family members. The challenge of effective long-term caring is to be close to the chronically ill person and at the same time distant.

When Cathy institutionalized her mother in the nursing home, she began the first steps of "easing off" or letting go. However, several issues made this difficult. The doctors had not expected her mother to survive the second stroke. The recovery was a surprise, and no one knew how long she would live or when she might have a heart attack or another stroke. Cathy began to prepare herself emotionally for her mother's death. Although she knew that she had done her best for her, she still felt overwhelming hurt and sadness at the prospect.

Cathy had hoped things would turn out differently. Daily phone conversations with her father hurt her a lot. He felt guilty— if only he had taken better care of her, he said, he should have been able to prevent the strokes. Listening to him cry was a shattering experience because Cathy had never known her father to cry. He had always maintained a tough exterior.

Letting go of parents is a complicated process. It is anchored in a fundamental fact of life: All of us are mortal, and eventually we will die. Letting go when parents are suffering and death is prolonged, however, is extraordinarily painful and difficult. Letting go often means more than distancing from or spending less time with the chronically ill parents. In different situations it takes different forms. For some people, letting go means "easing off" and spending less time. In other cases the time spent together does not change, but the caregiver's sense that they need to solve every single problem lessens. And in other situations it means finding outside help, day care, assisted care living, financial help, or even nursing home care.

Letting go thus involves changing expectations of yourself. Increasing separation from your aging, sick parents is essential if you and the rest of your family are to get on with life. This does not mean that you abandon your parents, but it does mean that you set limits on what you do. Families reorganize as generations are born, grow old, and die, and family members' responsibilities and commitments shift accordingly. What is ethically perplexing in these transitions is how to act responsibly toward those who are suffering chronic illnesses, while at the same time meeting other family needs.

Another issue involved in letting go is the desire of parents themselves to die. Many older persons, and even younger chronically ill individuals, prefer death to continuing a life of pain and suffering. Often they want to let go of life while the caregivers are still committed to keeping them alive and are fearful of death and separation.

As a society we have begun to appreciate the value of "death with dignity" and the problems associated with the use of extraordinary means, such as high-tech equipment, to extend people's functions when there is no quality to their existence. By regulation, older persons on Medicare are now routinely asked to indicate their wishes concerning life-sustaining strategies when they are admitted to hospitals. The issue is more complicated than just getting a signature, however. Family members need to know and respect the desires of the patient and be willing to support their expressed desires. Knowing that a parent died as they wished can be gratifying, even if life is somewhat shortened as a consequence. Maintaining quality of life includes controlling the quality of death.

GUIDELINES TO THE SEVEN STEPS

Before we launch into a detailed discussion of each of the seven steps and the many issues we have raised, we want to review several issues that it is important for you to keep in mind as you take on caregiving responsibilities.

1. *Chronic illnesses last a lifetime.* The challenges of aging and chronic illness can be overwhelming to caregivers, precisely because they impact upon virtually every aspect of life for a long time. While there is no "cookbook" with specific rules, there are many things you can do to prepare for what lies ahead of you in order to protect your finances, your health, your children, and your parents.

2. *Home is where the action is.* For most of us home is the place that makes us most comfortable. The Latin root of *comfortable—confortare*—means "to strengthen greatly." Although your parents may spend time in a hospital or other health care site, most of your caregiving exchanges will occur at home—theirs and yours.

3. Nursing homes can be homes. One of society's greatest challenges in long-term care is to provide a range of supportive community-based services to assist chronically ill people and their families. Nursing homes have a legitimate and important place in the spectrum of long-term care services. Even living at home can amount to a "one-person nursing home." Such home care, however, may compromise the health and well-being of you and your family if you refuse to relinquish a sick, impaired relative to others who are better able to provide the care needed.

Too often children promise "No, I'll never put you in a nursing home!" without thinking about the implications. These promises are usually made under duress, in some ways like fabled "shotgun weddings." Such promises should be reevaluated and reconsidered as something less than binding agreements based upon the careful and freely determined decision of capable consenting parties.

4. The responsibility for parent-caring is not the sole domain of adult children. Except when parents are severely mentally or physically impaired, they have responsibilities for their own health, safety, and well-being. Parents also have rights to privacy and autonomy—the rights to make decisions about themselves, their bodies, and their lives. Even when chronic illness impairs their health and safety, aging parents may still reject the intrusion of family or nonfamily support. As tough as it may be, unless extraordinary circumstances exist—such as sever dementia, depression, or paranoia (which can be determined with professional consultation)—your parents have the right to refuse your help.

This creates an extraordinary challenge for adult children. Parents need help but feel that to receive care is demeaning and degrading. The children may disagree, but for the parents, not getting intervention may be the more dignified alternative. Some people prefer to go out kicking and screaming rather than be institutionalized and coddled in a nursing home. Respecting these decisions is not easy, but in some cases it may be the right thing.

5. Living with chronic illness is hard work. Family members need to develop two styles of coping, both of which become increasingly difficult as time goes on. One is to develop coping strategies to deal with the needs of the chronically ill. Simple activities and routines may become extraordinarily demanding, both in energy and patience. Assisting sick parents with the daily activities of bathing and dressing, eating and drinking, even walking and toileting, may not only require hours but may be embarrassing for everyone.

The second style of coping is restructuring daily life routines to meet the needs of everyone else in the family. A reasonable quality of life requires a certain amount of freedom from caring for others. Creating opportunities for respite—time out—as well as programming other necessary activities—children, work, even leisure—may take a great deal of effort, but it is essential over the long haul.

6. *Your ability to cope with stress and uncertainty are the most precious resources you have.* Effective problem solving is the key to successfully meeting the challenges of daily routines through all phases of chronic illness. It takes money and energy, as well as emotional and physical endurance, to survive the seemingly interminable demands of caregiving.

In the early phases of a chronic illness families commonly spend a lot of time focused on the needs of the chronically ill person. If this intense activity continues for long periods, however, the needs of other family members will be neglected. A major objective associated with both coping and living is to define the wishes, needs, and preferences of everyone, including the recipient. This may even mean having everyone make a list on paper and then comparing notes. This can be a helpful exercise periodically, because it allows agreements and priorities to be made in an open manner. We are not suggesting that rational decision-making procedures will make parent-caring simple and easy. These strategies do, however, provide solid anchors in a future that often seems uncertain.

7. *Examine the limits of what you can do.* When parents are sick, incapacitated, or lonely, they have needs and expectations of how, when, and where people should respond to them. They may reject some needed help but they may also have unrealistic expectations about receiving other support. As one mother who wanted more

attention stated to her working daughter, who was also raising three children, "You'll have them forever, but you will only have me around a few more years."

A likely response of caregivers is to feel obligated to do what is expected of them, particularly if the expectation is voiced or even hinted at by their parents. Although meeting obligations over the short term may feel good or at least reduce guilt, meeting these extended obligations in an unqualified way over the long term may create anger and frustration, as well as many other reactions. This becomes a vicious cycle when other demands are ignored or postponed and pressures from children, spouse, and work increase relentlessly.

Under some circumstances it is important to recognize that although you can meet some or most of your parents' needs, you cannot always meet their expectations of how those needs are to be met. Sometimes parents' expectations are not even stated or are stated in a way that generates guilt: "I know that you are too busy to . . ." If your parents' expectations are beyond your resources but you have a reasonable plan of action, you must learn to accept that you have probably done the best you could under the circumstances. You may need to get someone to help you deal with your own unreasonable expectations of what you should be doing, or to resolve your dilemmas when a guilt-provoking parent makes unrealistic demands on you.

Sometimes it is legitimate not to feel obligated to meet someone's expectations. Anger and contempt toward parents are tough encumbrances for children to carry, but these feelings may be real and unresolvable. Recognizing your feelings and doing what you feel is appropriate is the best course to follow. It can be helpful in such cases to talk to another relative or friend to ensure that you are not merely hiding from your true feelings.

8. Caregiving interventions should be structured so that people make small successive adjustments rather than major adaptations. Most of the time, responding to the needs of chronically ill parents does not require emergency room life-or-death swiftness. Indeed, just the opposite is usually in order. Small changes and a slow, steady pattern of change are easier to manage than larger adaptations. It is also easier to understand small changes, since it gives you the time and space to renegotiate the many consequences of the changes for family relationships and obligations.

Developing a work plan with specific goals and a timetable will help you define the pattern of small successive changes needed. The plan should focus on the health and personal needs of the chronically ill individual, but when other family members are providing care, their desires and preferences also need to be integrated into the work plan and the timetable.

9. *If you have children, involve them.* Children, even young children, can sometimes be valuable partners in family caregiving. To exclude them can create a number of problems for them, such as the anxiety of not knowing what is wrong, or sadness or guilt that they are somehow responsible, or anger that they are being excluded or deprived by the loss of your attention.

Children are not empty containers. They are full of thoughts and feelings about what is going on. Like everyone else in the family, they have a legitimate right to be kept informed, to be allowed to express their feelings, and if possible to be involved in ways in which they are comfortable. Involving children also creates opportunities for you to spend time with them and teach them the value of caring for others. These bonds may give you the emotional support you need to deal with your own parents as well as strengthen the entire family.

LEARNING THE VALUE OF GROWING OLD

Children have long been regarded as society's most precious resources, and there is no doubt that our continuing civilization depends upon the success and well-being of the generations that follow. However, young children grow up to become adult children with their own children, who also grow up and grow old. Growing up and growing old are among life's greatest opportunities, and it is within the family that individuals learn how to master these challenges.

The rapidly increasing population of older people is creating significant pressures on adult children to find responsible ways to relate to their own children, their spouse, their parents, and to their personal needs. In the next centuries, when our descendants examine the end of the twentieth century and the beginning of the next millennium, they will find that the rapid aging of society caused a collision of values about caring and human life.

The following letter was written by one of our clients, David Jenson, to his brother Tommie. It reflects on his sick mother as well as emotional reactions to his family responsibilities:

Dear Tommie,

I don't know why I am writing this. I guess I needed to confide in someone. It feels strange to ask for help. You know how I have always been big brother to you and Sis. You two were always the ones coming to me with your problems. Everyone in the family has always come to me for practical advice, or to arbitrate difficult decisions and even for financial help. I was proud to be able to help.

I am not that person anymore. I wish there were a wall separating me from everything and everyone. I've failed with Mom—I can't seem to reach her anymore. Looking at her last week had all the clarity of a spotlight. She must go into a nursing home or move in with us, but she refused to do either.

Mom has wanted to die ever since Dad passed away. She won't eat properly or take care of herself. Now she even sounds a little confused. Whenever we speak, she repeatedly talks about dying. Our mother, who used to be so charming, witty, and energetic, is now fundamentally changed. It hurts to see her.

I am also angry that she is giving up. I remember how she nursed me back to health when I was just a young boy. Everyone, even the doctors, thought I would die—everyone, that is, except Mom; I was only four years old but I remember her, a colored blur, sitting by my bed. "You are a Jenson," she would say to me as she stroked my hair, "and every Jenson must do something remarkable before they die."

After I recovered, I remember thinking how I had to grow up and do something to make her proud of me. I cannot shake those memories now. I keep feeling that I must take care of her, but she won't let me and I am helpless.

Although his impulse was to take over and remake his mother's life as he wished it to be, David eventually decided to have his mother admitted to a nursing home in the town where she had lived for more than fifty years. He and his wife, Jane, flew in to visit her regularly for the next two months, before she died. At David's insistence, the entire family—brothers, sisters, aunts and uncles, nieces and nephews, and grandchildren—visited Mrs. Jenson, so that no weekend passed without some relative being with her. She died peacefully one afternoon while David was sitting at the bedside stroking her hair.

Weeks later, when David and Jane were cleaning out his mother's apartment, he found an old album from his parents' fiftieth wedding anniversary. Inside the album cover was a yellowed piece of lined paper with her handwriting. The words were familiar, part of a speech she had given at that anniversary party:

> As I have grown older, I see myself as fortunate in many ways. I have been privileged to witness my children and grandchildren become real people, each taking advantage of the endless possibilities of life. I have also experienced my own fierce pleasure to be and add what little I could to the world. Perhaps most of all I have been blessed with a passionate loving husband who has given me much joy.
>
> Our family is like a magical elixir. Each person is different, but when all together they form something boundlessly new. I pray we have many healthy, beautiful years together, and if either Joe or I become seriously ill, I pray we die quickly so the family can move on, reinvesting their love in the great-grandchildren yet to come. There are too many of us old folks around these days.

What did Mrs. Jenson mean by her last remark? Are there really too many "old folks," or are there too few people who understand the positive value of growing old while they focus on the negatives? Our society's precious heritage is its people of all ages. We are all guardians of each other's health and welfare, fiduciaries for our future and trustees of our most precious resource—ourselves and each other. The challenge that confronts us is to find ways we can play a positive role throughout our adult years and care for one another in the face of the unprecedented, rapid aging of our society.

We hope this book helps you meet this challenge. The next seven chapters describe the ways families come together or move apart as they reorganize around aging relatives. As we highlight the seven steps of change in different families, we recognize that we are chopping up the family ecology in order to focus on individual parts of what are really dynamic interactions. By attending to the stages of change and taking snapshots of family life, we can focus on specific issues and discuss strategies and tactics to achieve more effective caregiving.

1

RECOGNIZING AND PRIORITIZING PROBLEMS

Recognizing the problems that exist is the first step to successfully solving them. Identifying problems is not a static process. Numerous problems arise during caregiving as circumstances change, challenging caregivers to track the changes and alter their plans. Your ability to recognize problems will evolve as your knowledge increases and your perspective is enlarged. Your attitudes may even shift. It is much like reading a series of newspaper articles to follow an ongoing story, learning more details and gaining greater insights as the story unfolds.

Since effectivity as a caregiver depends on effective problem-solving, recognizing problems is an important skill to cultivate. This may sound simple and obvious, but it is not always easy to tell when something serious is happening to aging parents. Family members may not even know they need help. Many older people living into their eighties, nineties, or beyond become progressively frail and need some assistance but are too proud to ask for help from their children.

If parents have a condition such as heart disease, high blood pressure, arthritis, dementia, or diabetes—to list only a few—then their problem is clearly a health problem. A heart attack or a fall and broken hip will precipitate an emergency visit to the hospital—again, an obvious problem. But recognizing other problems of aging parents may be far more complicated than this. Young and old people alike commonly deny that anything is wrong, and older people often shrug their own symptoms off as just the result of growing old. Even if aging parents are getting medical help, they may not be diagnosed accurately. Or they may have multiple physicians, each of whom is taking charge of an isolated problem and prescribing medications, unaware of what the others are doing.

This chapter is intended to help you "see" what is happening to your aging parents. Independent of the specific condition involved, there are five factors that affect your ability to recognize problems:

- You and your view of the world
- Your fear of aging
- Your knowledge about aging and health problems
- Your motivation to care
- The way your family works

You and Your View of the World

Your self-knowledge is a critical component in your ability to recognize problems. Lasting solutions to parent-caring problems will come only when you are able to understand how you think and feel about yourself. Your view of yourself affects the way you see other people as well. In turn, until you come to grips with how you see yourself and others, you will not be able to understand how others see and feel about themselves. If you are not aware of the connections between how you see yourself and how you see others, you risk projecting your own feelings and beliefs about your parents onto them. When a disagreement arises, you will believe that you are being objective and they are not.

Numerous studies show that the feelings people attribute to others can be mirrors of their own feelings and be only minimally related to the actual state of the other person. If you tend to be overly optimistic, for example, you are likely to discount the problems your parents talk about as being of little significance. You will simply not believe that your parents could have problems. A reservoir of resentment and anger toward your parents, on the other hand, can lead to you believing that their expressions of pain and need are merely their usual whining or chronic complaining. Your attitude of pessimism or guilt may cause you to mentally exaggerate every problem, ache, or pain they have, and you will treat them as children who need to be managed rather than as adults. A fear of sickness and death on your part can lead to excessive reliance on physicians and hospitals or, conversely, to a rejection of professionals as having no value.

Your views and feelings about your parents' condition are also influenced by the nature of the relationship you have had with them. If your parents caused you great pain over the years, you may still feel you owe them care and respect simply because they are your parents. At the same time, you may feel anger and resentment toward them. Knowing yourself means recognizing and accepting a range of feelings as legitimate, and then getting beyond them. If you focus on your negative feelings toward your parents and how they hurt you in the past, you may feel victimized and therefore be unable to mobilize yourself to do anything constructive. If you want your parents to be more cooperative and to work more effectively with you, you should take the initiative and try to be more cooperative with them.

Recognizing your own feelings may be as simple as listening to yourself when you talk about your parents. It is important to allow yourself to feel and not try to deceive yourself about your feelings. It can be helpful to get a spouse or good friend to listen uncritically to your comments about your situation, and if you can, listen to their impressions of what you said without feeling resentful or guilty about their observations. It is essential that you not blame the mirror for what you see in it. It may be useful to tape-record what you say to others when you are discussing your parents. You can then play the conversation back and listen to yourself, to the tone of your speech as well as to what you say.

Self-help groups for people with such disorders as Alzheimer's disease, heart disease, cancer, and many others can be helpful. If your feelings are too much for you to handle, mental health centers and mental health professionals are valuable resources. If you cannot talk about your situation without crying, getting uncontrollably angry, blaming someone, or feeling that the future is hopeless and that you are helpless to do anything, professional help is probably necessary. Dealing with these emotions is the focus of Chapter 3.

Your Fear of Aging

Whether adult children's relationships with parents are good or bad, watching them change with age, become disabled, or die forces a confrontation with the illusion of immortality. Aging and death cease to be abstractions. Even when parents age in good health, the many physical changes are a reminder to their children that time is passing, triggering questions and anxieties about the future. Most people are emotionally unprepared to see their parents grow old and die.

Confronting the realities of increasing frailty, chronic illness, and death reminds people of what lies ahead not only for their parents but for themselves. Many people do not like to think or talk about being old. Most are afraid of aging and try to avoid dealing with it—they even lie about their age. It is this fear and avoidance that often interferes with the ability to recognize their older parents' situation and understand them as human beings.

Ivan Williams, a fifty-two-year-old man caring for both of his parents, writes about this fear.

> Long before the heart attack, I could see Mom and Dad were changing. They were growing older, and it upset me.
>
> I loved them and enjoyed their company, but the wrinkles upset me . . . not the wrinkles themselves, but what they represented. I knew less time was ahead of them than behind.
>
> I didn't want them to grow old, and I didn't want to lose them. I even had crazy thoughts that they would live forever. I knew this was magical thinking.

My fears also kept me from seeing another side of my parents. As we got closer I saw that Dad was more than an ambitious driven businessman—the person I knew as a child . . . He was an ambitious driven person about everything! This man saw every second as a window of opportunity. In his seventies, he translated a book, won several photographic awards, went to Europe, and sponsored two foster children. Even Mom didn't know about all of his awards. He was too embarrassed because two years in a row he won first, second, and third place!

Most of us go through life unaware of the exact date we will die. However, as the years go by, there comes a time when, short of an accident or premature death, our bodies remind us that we are no longer young. In his book *The Orphaned Adult*, Rabbi Marc Angel tells the story of a young man who had a dream in which God appeared and granted him the opportunity for one wish. The young man did not want to die suddenly. He asked God to give him a warning, and God agreed.

The years passed, and the young man grew old and gray. Finally, one night he passed away in his sleep. When he arrived in heaven, the man was angry and demanded an audience with God. He accused God of forgetting his promise because he had died in his sleep with no warnings.

But God replied he had kept his promise, and that he had given the man many warnings!

The man objected furiously, but God simply replied: "Look at your gray hair, your wrinkled skin, the way you bend when you walk, and how easily tired you become. I gave you many warnings, but you did not pay attention!"

As people age there are many signs, and most of us, at some point, encounter an event or set of circumstances that forces us to pay attention to the fact that we are not as young as we used to be. Juan Alvarez described the first time he realized he himself was getting older:

I first thought about my own aging the week I stayed with Mom when Dad went into the hospital. I had to take care of her round the clock. I fed her, administered medications, walked her like a child, and listened to her groans of pain all night.

The second night Mom needed help in the bathroom—she couldn't sit without my holding her, and she needed help wiping herself. Tears streamed down her face. I did what I had to do and also gently wiped the tears away—hers and mine.

Later when I washed my hands, I couldn't stop looking at all the wrinkles. My hands were no longer those of a young man. My hands and I had aged!

Most of us have much to learn about how to conquer our fears about aging and much to discover about what it means to have meaningful and productive years. We may have important lessons to learn from our parents, and they often occur when we least expect them, as Larry Chang, a thirty-nine-year-old business-man, describes:

At first Dad and Mom were furious about my suggestion that they move to a retirement community. When Thanksgiving rolled around, they even refused to celebrate with us. However, the night before, we drove to their place and sent all the grand-children to the door to ask them to join us for Thanksgiving dinner. They had to accept!

At dinner Dad joked and teased Alissa, the youngest of the brood. He hadn't been this outgoing since before his heart at-tack. After dinner we adjourned to the living room where he enthralled her with his version of the story of Dorothy and the land of Oz as we sat having coffee. Alissa clutched him tightly as he spoke of the Wicked Witch, and we all laughed at his funny imitations of the Tin Man, the Cowardly Lion, and the Scarecrow.

That sight brought a lump to my throat. I saw that Dad still brought magic into the world. In my daughters's eyes he was safety and comfort for her fears, and he was still the one who gave continuity to our family. Did he understand how much all of us needed him and Mom as part of our family?

This moment of reflection captures one of the challenges of later life—to recognize that we have a meaningful place in society and in the family. A major function of the family has always been to shelter its members. Belonging to a family carries membership privileges regardless of a person's accomplishments, and the special role of being parents, grandparents, or great-grandparents provides irretrievable opportunities to contribute to the lasting emotional well-being of the entire family. Older generations not only teach values and nurture the young, but by their very existence they involve family members in social situations that will leave a permanent imprint on future generations.

Our own children learn a lot from watching us with our parents, especially when help is needed. How we reorganize family life to care for and love our aging parents becomes a legacy that our children witness and integrate into their lives. Through our own actions we teach them what is appropriate and what is worth making sacrifices for. Children need to experience the family as a safe, protective environment for everyone, not just themselves, and to see the rewards of giving when it is appropriate for everyone's collective welfare. Larry Chang recalls that his daughter Alissa interrupted a family argument with a poignant statement that made everyone realize that the argument was hurtful and unnecessary:

> We met after Sunday dinner to review the financial considerations of the many retirement communities we had seen. Dad and Mom wanted to go to a modest condominium close by that had a refundable endowment fee if they died or moved out within a year.
>
> My brother and sister argued that they should go to a fancier community without the refund in a warmer climate because they owed it to themselves. It was their money. They should spend it on themselves and not worry about leaving it for the kids. But Mom and Dad were adamant about leaving a financial legacy.
>
> At one point everyone stormed out of the room frustrated and angry. Dad headed for the bathroom while Mom and I made coffee. When we brought the coffee and snacks back into the living room, we met an unexpected sight.
>
> Alissa was sitting on the couch next to Dad. Her little arms were crossed and her face was set in a strong scowl: "I heard you

fighting and I know how to settle everything. Here is my bank-
book! I want Grandpa and Grandma to have it. Then no one
will have to fight about money!"

Aging parents and grandparents play an important role in preparing those who are younger for a future that ultimately includes
death. Larry Chang was eventually successful in helping his parents move into a retirement community, and they thrived with
new friends and new opportunities. One afternoon Larry's father
humorously announced to his children that he and his wife would
die soon because this new lifestyle was too fast and would burn
them out! Humorous comments like these were a way Larry's parents prepared him to understand that death was, according to his
father, "only the completion of being . . . like the sun setting after
a long day." Larry wrote:

> Dad jokes about dying to prepare me, even though I don't want
> to hear it. He says accepting death is like taking a train ride on a
> route with many stops. He knows that this stop is the last one
> and at some point he must do the inevitable—get off!

Every generation prepares for its own future in the way it cares
for older persons. William F. Woo, editor of the *St. Louis Post-
Dispatch*, wrote a column describing how values and behaviors are
shaped from generation to generation. He referred to a story of
filial piety depicted on a sixth-century Chinese sarcophagus in the
Nelson Gallery in Kansas City, Missouri. The story underlines
children's duty to and respect for their parents, which Confucius
considered the highest of virtues:

> A man and his young son and also an old man [are] sitting on a
> pallet. The family does not have enough food, so the father and
> son are carrying the grandfather to the woods. There they leave
> him to die.
> As they return, the man asks: "But why are you bringing
> the pallet home, my son?" The boy replies: "Because, Father,
> someday we shall use it for you."

Your Knowledge About Aging and Health Problems

Aging is not a disease. But as people grow older, the risks are greater that a number of health problems will complicate the aging process. Across American society, life expectancy has increased in recent decades, but the major killers—cardiovascular disease, cerebrovascular disease or stroke, and cancer—often cripple people long before they kill them. Arthritis, for example, is the leading cause of disability, but conditions like hearing loss, visual impairment, depression, Alzheimer's disease and related disorders, hypertension, and diabetes all affect the quality of later life. They can make aging a bitter curse rather than a blessing.

Many of these diseases appear with different symptom patterns in later life. A heart attack, for example, is not always accompanied by severe chest pain. An older person who is depressed may not act sad and cry but may show physical symptoms such as increased pain, fatigue, weight loss, or weight gain, and they may withdraw from social activities. Furthermore, the treatment of these disorders and conditions with medications can also cause side effects that mimic other diseases.

There are a number of useful books (see Selected Readings) that can help you spot health problems in older relatives. These books are intended to educate you about common symptoms and conditions. None of them should replace the judgment and involvement of competent health professionals willing to take the time to do an evaluation and explain the results.

The appearance of any unusual sign or symptom—physical, mental, or emotional—merits a visit to the doctor, because a correct diagnosis is the first step in proper treatment. Since older persons usually have several coexisting conditions and are using several medications, proper medical care to insure their optimal functioning may involve coordinating the activities of a number of specialists. This may be one of your more interesting challenges.

Older people are not really different from younger people—they are only much more complicated! Contrary to mythology, most older adults respond well to appropriate surgery and other treatments. Neglecting to consult trained professionals can mean risking a range of difficulties—an incorrect diagnosis and improper treatment, unnecessary pain and suffering, creating new problems, and even an early death! A well-trained family physician, internist, or psychiatrist, especially one qualified in geriatrics, can play a major role in helping you and can be one of your best partners in caring. How to approach health professionals and work with them effectively is the subject of Chapter 4.

Your Motivation to Care

The way you see the needs of your aging parents is often affected by your motivation to care. Your motivation has an important impact on your willingness to do the job of caring for them and the degree to which you are willing to become involved with it. Helping dependent aging parents is often motivated by many forces, but there are six particularly powerful ones: love, equity, morality, ethics, envy, and greed. You may be influenced by one or more of these forces, and it is not uncommon for all of them to affect your behavior.

Love. It is impossible to calculate or even adequately describe the feeling of love that exists between children and their parents, but it can be reflected in part by the feelings of loss and sadness that persist well after a parent dies. Love is a unique force that motivates people to extend themselves in caring.

Love is a powerful emotion. Because it has so many facets and is directed in so many different ways, it is difficult to measure and can have many meanings. Love can mean being closely tied to another person by affection, commitment, intimacy, passion, or faith. However, there are other ways to think of love. M. Scott Peck in *The Road Less Traveled* describes love as a form of work, involving commitment and a conscious effort to make decisions and take actions.

We also express love in different ways toward the various people who are important to us. Love for a child is a powerful emotion, and some studies indicate that animal mothers will endure the greatest pain to help their offspring. The love of a man and woman can be strong enough to break strong family ties, as described in *Fiddler on the Roof,* where Tevye tries to hold on to his love of tradition and religion while he also tries to understand his daughter, whose love for her husband causes her to leave the family. Friendship powerful enough that a man lays down his life for others in a battle is yet another form of love. And the love of God is among the most potent forces in our world. Love can be powerful and irrational, and you cannot ignore it as you examine your caregiving plans.

Equity. Family members often report a sense of owing their parents something: "My mother took care of me when I was young, and I couldn't live with myself if I didn't take care of her now that she is sick and needs me." Our need to express equity or reciprocity by paying our parents back for their years of care and nurturance (or neglect and indifference) of us plays an important role in our approach to caring for them in later years. Reciprocity may be related to love, but it is a separate motivation as well.

When parent-child relationships have been unpleasant, distant, or hurtful, it is common for the adult children to wonder, "Why should I help him? He was never there when I needed him." Such caregivers may feel bitter and resentful when they do help because in part their true inclination is to ignore the parents and walk away.

Equity means doing something because we believe it to be fair and just. What is fair and just is a personal decision, and others may disagree with your reckoning. Your husband, wife, or friend may say, "Enough is enough," and there may be considerable merit to their position. However, your own feelings of responsibility are what count in such a decision. Each of us assesses the value of what our parents gave us and the repayment that we need to make for the relationship to be an equitable one. Clearly, most parents give to children without real concern for eventual—if any—return. Some children appreciate what was done; some denigrate it; and some overvalue it. Many feel that repayment for parental help involves giving support to the next generation rather than to the parents themselves. Equity as a motivation is undeniable and should be explicit in your care equation.

Morality. Morality, another complex motivational force, is a code of conduct reflecting a society's principles of right and wrong and the awareness of what is expected of people. Statements like "You can't leave your father alone!" and "How could you allow your mother to live in such awful conditions?" reflect a society's moral code. Personal morality involves a conscious awareness of what others will say and a need to do what is proper in the social setting.

While it may appear to have more form than substance, doing what is expected is a strong factor in this and every society. Society, however, may expect more of you than you wish or are able to give, and your fear of embarrassment can place you in a position which you find untenable. Occasionally persons with a vested interest will play on this embarrassment to influence you. A funeral director, for example, may pressure you into purchasing a more expensive casket, so that your neighbors will not see you as cheap and uncaring. Individuals themselves may pin their pride and "self-respect" on how well they conform to the perceived morality of their culture, and their fear of violating social expectations can drive them to extremes they may otherwise wish to avoid.

Ethics. An inner sense of what is right often intuitively guides our actions. "My father was a selfish, miserly person who abused me physically when I was a kid, but he is in bad shape now and there's no one else to help him," you may reason. "I guess it's up to me to make sure he is placed in a decent nursing home and gets adequate care. I don't want or need to visit him. I just want to make sure that he is getting what any human being deserves."

Ethics is what people have learned to believe is the right thing to do for one another. It consists of a combination of personal beliefs and assimilated social expectations, encouraging us to conform to the norms of the community in which we live. Our own various ethical values may also conflict with each other. Parents and children born in different times and cultures may have different expectations of what is right or wrong, and responsibilities for providing care for your parents could conflict with your responsibilities for caring and educating your children. Such ethical dilemmas are among the most difficult to resolve.

Envy. Some motivations for taking care of parents are more negative than love, ethics, and morality. Envy is a complex motivating force that can take several different forms. Some adult children may envy their parents' material possessions, for instance, but more commonly, envy operates in a different way.

Many adult children envy the love and respect their parents seem to feel for their siblings. As parents age and need help, children may try to earn their parents' love and respect by outdoing their siblings in caregiving. Sibling rivalry can thereby reach new levels of competitiveness. As if reenacting childhood fantasies of control, children may seek to "capture" their parents' affection by outdoing their siblings in goodness.

If competitiveness among siblings envious of one another's close relationships with their parents is not recognized and dealt with, it can lead to divisive, even destructive, conflict. A "holier than thou" attitude can reach absurdity on the level of "I'm humbler than anyone I know." Even if extremely competitive children achieve the parental love and respect they seek, they do so without fulfillment, since their motivation is negative.

Greed. Finally, an expectation of material gain may be a driving force for caring. Although most adult children will not talk about this easily, their desire to be in line for family assets can make some individuals willing caregivers, and it can make others jealous and vicious toward other family members. Such fractious behavior often continues after the parents' death, and legal battles over estates are not unusual, although almost always they are catastrophic to the families involved.

Concern for parental assets is not always greed. It can be a genuine concern to control the expenses associated with the costs of care. Sometimes we are less concerned about a legacy than about the prospect of a financial burden, merely hoping that "things will come out even." On occasion, however, caring can be compromised by the desire to preserve the estate for the "next generation." This happens when the expenses for caring are restricted, to the detriment of the parents' best interests. Sibling conflict or intergenerational criticism should not be dismissed as a factor when these issues emerge.

Love, equity, morality, ethics, envy, and greed—all are powerful forces in family relationships, even though we usually do not readily analyze our behavior in these terms. These motivations have a profound impact on what we do for ourselves and other people. And they are not independent of one another. It is human to experience all these motivations. The challenge is to recognize and figure out how they affect your own ability to understand and deal with your aging parents' problems.

THE WAY YOUR FAMILY WORKS

When an older parent experiences difficulties, the family system must respond in some way. This response will depend partly on how family members have treated one another in the past. The response to parental dependency will set up certain family behavior patterns as adult children and other family members become incorporated into the decision-making process. If you are not aware of these behavior patterns, you will be sucked into the process without identifying your family's most significant problems.

In families in which a particular pattern of decision making and problem-solving evolves, certain behaviors and styles of decision making are characteristic of the "family way" of doing things. David Reiss, a family researcher, has described this family way of doing things as a "family paradigm." This paradigm is the set of beliefs and rules by which the family and its members characteristically deal with the world. This paradigmatic way of doing things can interfere with recognizing problems if a person does not understand the family.

The case of the Farber family illustrates what we mean. Bernie and Lois Farber, both in their seventies, had been married for fifty-two years. They lived in the same community with their five children—three girls and two boys—and their families. The Farbers were a close-knit group and regularly spent time with their children and grandchildren. The two sons were part of the family business that Bernie had established and continued to run until he died after a sudden heart attack.

Bernie had run the business from their home, which had enabled him to be Lois's constant companion. They had a strong marriage, friendship, and partnership. Indeed, Lois had been the "silent partner" behind her husband's success, even though she had been severely crippled for many years by arthritis. Bernie's business had thrived with her entrepreneurial drive and advice. Despite being crippled and in pain most of the time, Lois had channeled her energy into shaping the business, but in a way that supported her husband. After his death, it remained to be seen how she would exercise authority and guidance in business with the boys.

In spite of her grief, Lois talked openly with her children and grandchildren about her need for the family to get on with its life. She had long been the emotional and decision-making center of family life, and she maintained that control even more openly after Bernie's death. Lois invited her sons to take over the business and then announced that if all went well, she would relinquish financial control to them over the next year. About three months later, she asked an old friend, also recently widowed, to move in with her as a companion who would live with and assist her.

Lois Farber's inner strength transcended her disability both before and after her husband's death. She was an energetic woman who inspired her family and everyone around her to enjoy life and meet adversity head on. Although the family was organized around her strong identity, she orchestrated the rhythm of family and community life in a way that generated a common concern for everyone's welfare. The Farber family was an intimate group whose central beliefs were invested in an active, independent family life. Problems were identified and solved, heavily orchestrated by the maternal control of Lois Farber.

The problems of aging parents turn life upside down in every family. It is a fact of life! Although the nature and severity of parents' needs will vary—from death and chronic illness, as in the Farber family, to a temporary incapacitation, such as minor surgery and a hospital stay—the initial response of virtually every family is the same—to rearrange everyday routines to accommodate what has happened. The important issue here is to recognize what you and your family are doing. Some family paradigms adapt easily to crises. Change and flexibility are part of the family pattern, and explicit rules and behaviors vary according to perceived needs. Other families are rigid and inflexible, decision making is not shared, and the rules of succession are unclear. For such families, adapting to change, particularly when the parents become impaired, is a crisis. Although things may go along smoothly at first, the system breaks down with increasing need for a flexible response.

During the early phases of a crisis, implicit rules of behavior are established, based upon the family's usual ways of helping members come to grips with a problem. These rules or adjustments in family behavior may be effective in the beginning, but they often must be changed as time goes on. As the problems become more complicated, recognition becomes a continuing process of tracking and responding. We illustrate how new family rules get established in the following stories involving the Gonzalez and the Shelby families.

Mrs. Gonzalez, age seventy-two, fell off the kitchen stool one day while reaching for some canned goods. She struck her head on the sink and suffered a massive hemorrhage. Unfortunately, she died shortly after being admitted to the hospital. Her husband was on a fishing trip in the Canadian wilderness at the time. When Mr. Gonzalez returned to discover the tragedy, he went into a profound depression. In this period of acute grief his daughter and son-in-law developed a simple rule: "Someone in the family must always be with Dad." This reflects the paradigm of a close, supportive family. The purpose of this rule was to help Mr. Gonzalez deal with the shock of his wife's sudden death. He was obsessed with guilt about being away when she died, and the family was concerned about his talk of suicide.

The emergence of unspoken or explicit rules following a stressful event reveals a great deal about how the family system is changing and adjusting or not adapting. Prior to her accident, Mrs. Gonzalez had enjoyed an active lifestyle with her husband. Both were in excellent health and had traveled extensively together with their children and grandchildren for years. The daughter's plan to keep Mr. Gonzalez company provided a rule consistent with the family paradigm, whose core beliefs focused on family togetherness and enjoyment of the outdoors. Everyone seemed willing to be with Grandpa for as long as it took him to come to grips with the situation and get on with his life.

Over time, however, the Gonzalez family found that circumstances caused them to develop several more rules to guide them through the future, such as "Grandpa should be allowed to have some private space" and "Grandpa should spend weekends hunting or fishing with his buddies, or visiting with one of us." After six months Mr. Gonzalez seemed to have successfully dealt with his grief, and although the family continued to spend time together, the explicit rules were no longer necessary. The grandchildren were greatly relieved, especially the teenagers, who were beginning to resent the "grandpa-sitting" roles that took them away from their friends and social activities.

A different situation occurred in the Shelby family. The Shelbys were a three-generation family living on a farm. They too had a set of beliefs focused on family togetherness. One afternoon, Grandpa Shelby, who had Parkinson's disease, insisted on helping his sons. He lost his footing, fell, and suffocated in the grain elevator. It was hours before his body was discovered, and the horror of his death unnerved the entire family. After the funeral the family developed a pattern of behavior motivated by fear that someone else might be killed. The implicit rule became "No member of the family should leave the house alone!"

The rule was a natural outgrowth of the family style of togetherness and concern for one another. Before Grandpa Shelby was killed in the accident, everyone in the family had already worked long and hard hours together. The basic style of the family was that of a large intimate group who shared the farm tasks but also respected each person's privacy. After the grandfather's untimely death, instead of functioning smoothly as a community the family became preoccupied with their tragedy. The adults were particularly concerned that the children might get hurt, and the children were upset by the restrictions their parents imposed. Both parents and children were deeply concerned about Grandma Shelby, whom they would hardly allow to leave the house at all.

While the Gonzalez family gradually recovered from their grief, the Shelbys had more difficulty. What had once been a warm, congenial household now became angry and tense. Arguments, which had previously been rare, became the norm. Several of the children were truant from school, and Grandma Shelby became depressed and withdrawn, spending days at a time in bed. As a result of her absence, another rule emerged: "All the children are responsible for their own supper." This rule appeared to be benign, designed to teach the children a lesson in responsibility. But it had the unfortunate consequence that Grandma Shelby sometimes missed an evening meal if she stayed in bed. This in turn caused blame and guilt, escalating the arguments within the family.

After several weeks another rule emerged: "The children are not to make any more demands on their parents or Grandma." This rule had the potential to cause even more serious problems. A child could not go out alone in the evening and could not ask an adult. The child could leave the house only if Mr. or Mrs. Shelby or Grandma *initiated* the idea. Soon many upsetting events began to happen. The younger children refused to go to school, and the older children ignored their homework assignments. The oldest son even stayed out all night on a date without calling, upsetting everyone!

What emerged in the Shelby family as a direct result of their inconsistent and unreasonable family rules was a series of *maladaptive* behaviors that only increased tensions in the family. No one wanted to recognize their own responsibility in creating the unrealistic rules. Conflict became the norm since parents and children blamed each other for what was happening. Grandma Shelby threatened to move into an "old people's home." She blamed herself for what was happening to the family and at the same time accused her daughter and son for letting things get "out of control" and not being good parents.

The emergence of new rules or family patterns reveals a great deal about how well a family recognizes and addresses its problems. The degree to which family rules are inflexible, unable to effectively deal with the problems, contradict each other, or break old useful patterns is what leads to conflict. The disruptions in the Shelby family are an example of what happens when family rules are unrealistic and interfere with each other, while the smooth transition in the Gonzalez family illustrates the outcome of consistent family rules that adapt to changing circumstances.

As ongoing disruption of normal family routines during parent care leads to the establishment of more and more rules of behavior, conflict often emerges among the several members trying to dictate rules. This inevitably disrupts the family paradigm unless family members figure out what the rules are and how they are affecting people. It is valuable for family members to be sensitive to changes in mood in one another, particularly in the children, who may mirror what is happening as they play out unspoken tensions.

Therefore, one of the challenges in identifying problems is to discover what rules have been established in the family and whether they make sense to everyone. The next challenge is to decide to what extent new rules that have been developed to care for older parents should take priority over previously established rules that govern the rest of the family. As time goes on, some rules may stay the same and some will need to be adapted or added. It is when the rules conflict with each other that life gets unbalanced.

A common belief in parent-caring is "I must do everything for my mother or father." By definition, if this belief becomes a rule, it has the potential to conflict with every other rule of family life. The feeling of wanting to do "everything" is legitimate, but the actions associated with the feeling are usually impossible to carry out. If this rule continues to take priority and the demands for care are major, serious problems will emerge sooner or later unless you have unlimited resources.

Marcia and Jim Langer were intimately involved in caring for Marcia's mother, Mrs. Kurtz, who was living in a nursing home.

Their frequent visits to the nursing home were as much a part of their life as eating, breathing, working, and sleeping. When Mrs. Kurtz entered the nursing home, the Langers also paid for several private aides, an expense that cut deeply into their savings. In time the Langers had to dismiss all but one aide. Even one person was difficult for them to pay for, but they could not bring themselves to let the last aide go. To cut their own costs, Marcia and Jim decided to forgo their summer vacation, and Marcia set up a strict monthly budget. They stopped going out to eat, and Marcia took a second part-time job. Only when Jim came down with a severe case of hepatitis was Marcia forced to confront how much her mother's care dominated their entire life!

Marcia conveyed her desperation in the following letter to her cousin:

> I love my mother. I don't want her to die—but I want her to die. The stomach cancer is wasting her away, and she lingers on in such pain. She is a living skeleton now, held together by a yellow housedress.
>
> I know that Barbara is a comfort to her. When I'm there I can see how Mom looks at her. Barbara holds her hand and reads to her. I don't want Mom to be alone.
>
> Jim is very sick. He needs me and I spend less time visiting Mom. I'm also scared because I don't know how to keep paying Barbara. I'm caught between two people I love. I just feel helpless and out of control of my life.

Marcia was so distraught that it never occurred to her to ask her cousin or other family members to help. The rule "Help Mom at all costs" had become "*I* must help Mom at all costs." So powerful was this rule that Marcia became trapped in a spiral of increasing pressures, isolation, and financial impoverishment. Fortunately, Marcia's cousin recognized the problem and got other family members involved—at least for the period of Jim's illness.

The Langers' story is not unusual. It illustrates the importance of understanding the challenges that may create new problems in caring for aging parents. But you can control the way your life changes by understanding these problems and the need to take charge of the rules. Your plan should involve reformulating a series of explicit and realistic rules that you and your family can implement together.

The next chapter introduces you to the effects of denial. Just as people begin to see the problems that lie ahead, it is not unusual to deny they really exist.

2

OVERCOMING DENIAL

When my mother was dying I would lie in bed at night and imagine that she was not only well but a young woman again. I would close my eyes and pretend that she would live forever.

Amanda Thomas did not want to believe that her mother was dying—that the cancer would kill her. Although she and the rest of the family were very attentive, at night in the darkness of her room it was important for her to pretend that her mother was young and well. Pretending kept the anxiety away so that she could fall asleep. If Amanda could continue to see her mother as young, then in her mind at least, that would keep her mother from dying.

The fear of death may not be universal, but it arouses feelings in most of us. Consciously or unconsciously we may deny illness and death. And death is not the only fact we deny. As a matter of routine we continually filter information to avoid being over-whelmed and to escape hearing about anything we do not want to accept. The process of denial distorts unwanted facts, events, or feelings, revising them to partial truths or nontruths, or eliminates them altogether.

When our aging parents are sick, it can be very difficult for us to look at them, be close to them, or touch them. When people are in a hospital or nursing home, any number of conditions—matted hair, dry scaly skin, saliva, foul smells, soiled clothes—can create terrifying feelings. Just the sight of a frail, pale, hurting person in an institutional bed can be alarming. When our parents grow old in good health, the many changes in their bodies are a reminder to us that time is passing, triggering thoughts about what the future might hold for ourselves as well as for them. It is hard to face, let alone accept, that parents will eventually die or may live with a painful illness for a long time.

Six Signs of Denial

Denial is a natural reaction to shocking or unpleasant events. Whether it is the trauma of a car accident, a rape, a serious health condition, or the death of a loved one, it can have a paralyzing and numbing impact. The mind reacts to such events by sealing itself off and rejecting the notion that anything so awful could happen.

Throughout life, denial is an almost universal response to hurtful changes. To a certain degree, refusing to see that anything is wrong is adaptive behavior, especially when events occur over which people have no control. In a sense, the denial acts as a buffer, giving a person time to absorb the full impact of an upsetting experience or shock. Your denial is therefore helpful at first, allowing you to get over the shock and confront the pain. But then when you work through the denial, it hurts because you have to deal with the situation and your deeper feelings. This takes time and much effort, and most people need help from others to do it.

Psychologist Mardi Horowitz has described six signs of denial that occur when people are in distress:

1. *Your attention changes.* When you feel threatened and deny what is happening, your ability to perceive and attend to the world around you is affected. You may feel as if you are in a daze, that you are easily distracted, uncomfortable, ill at ease, and unable to appreciate what is going on around you.

2. *Your level of consciousness changes.* You may feel as if you are not really functioning at work, school, or home. You go through the

motions, doing things with little awareness of what you are doing or what is going on around you. You may not even remember many events that have occurred. It is not unusual to experience partial or complete amnesia for significant blocks of time.

3. Your ability to think and process information changes. You may concoct fantasies to explain what happened to you. You may lose your connection with reality and misinterpret what others say and do. You may become less efficient. Relatively simple tasks can appear very complicated. It is not unusual to obsess about the smallest action and be afraid to take on larger responsibilities.

4. Your emotions are blocked. You may not lose awareness of what has happened to you, but you may block out or alter your feelings and think about the event or problem in a highly intellectual fashion. You do not express how you feel but refer to the situation as if it were someone else's problem. You act in a mechanical way, hiding feelings that may emerge in more insidious ways later. Emotional blunting may occur, or you may explode easily, losing your temper over small, unrelated problems.

5. You feel aches and pains. Many people develop a variety of somatic problems but do not recognize that these bodily symptoms are the result of emotional reactions to emotional distress. It is not uncommon to have chest pains, headaches, skin rashes, and stomach problems and still deny that anything is wrong.

6. Your behavior changes. It is common to become obsessed with retreating or running away from the situation. You avoid activities such as visiting the hospital or nursing home or doing anything that brings you into contact with whatever situation has overwhelmed you.

Overcoming denial is not only basic to your effectiveness as a caregiver, it plays a role in your own physical and mental health. Therefore, learning to recognize the six signs of denial is important, and you may wish to review this section again from time to time. Recognizing denial is by definition difficult because it means you must confront something when you do not want to recognize or deal with it. We hope this chapter gives you the opportunity to look at yourself and think about what you are doing. Reading about the six signs of denial and discussing them with a friend or confidante should help you evaluate your behavior.

What Happens When Denial Continues

In most cases denial works itself out over the short run. In time, you will begin to mobilize yourself to overcome it. Denial can be harmful, however, if it prevents you from getting appropriate help for yourself or someone else in your family. As we said, denial acts as a shock absorber. When something goes wrong or hurts you, it is a cushion to protect you until you can mobilize yourself. If denial impedes you from eventually taking appropriate actions, it can hurt.

Sometimes professional help is important in working through denial. The following story of a mother and daughter illustrates the importance of getting help. It is not possible to review every aspect of their denial, but Marilyn and Abigail's story is intended as a case history with teaching value. As you read, think about them and then consider your circumstances. The message is not that everybody needs professional help. It is that unless you appreciate the potency of denial, you may get into trouble. If you know about it, at least you will be prepared.

Marilyn Haber was living through an exasperating summer. Her mother, Abigail Marcus, was driving her crazy with phone calls day and night starting about a month after Mrs. Marcus had had minor surgery. Marilyn's mother, who had always been so "with it," had changed into a demanding and fearful old woman. Mrs. Marcus complained about aches and pains all over her body, and she wanted Marilyn to visit her every day. She said she was afraid of living alone—although she had been alone quite successfully for the twelve years since her husband, Harry, had died.

A visit to her internist, Dr. Davies, after the surgery showed that Mrs. Marcus had recovered in record time and that at seventy-nine she was in excellent physical health. Throughout the examination she talked with Dr. Davies about her new grandchild in Ohio and her plans to visit her sister in California. She denied being upset or afraid, and she said that her daughter was exaggerating the number of phone calls she was making.

A week after the visit to the doctor, the phone calls increased to eight or ten times a day. Marilyn used an answering machine at home and instructed her secretary to take messages at work. She phoned her mother once in the morning and again each evening hoping to stop the calls, but to no avail. Marilyn asked her brother and sister in Ohio to call several times a week, but the calls from her mother continued.

One night Mrs. Marcus called Marilyn at two in the morning, demanding that she come over. Her heart was racing, and Mrs. Marcus was afraid that it was a heart attack. Marilyn rushed her mother to the emergency room, but the doctors found nothing. Dr. Davies recommended that Mrs. Marcus see a social worker.

At the first appointment several days later, Marilyn was surprised that her mother talked so openly about her fears with the social worker. For one thing, Mrs. Marcus was afraid of being a survivor. No one else in the family had lived this long, and she did not know what to expect. She was also afraid of becoming a burden.

Most of the important people in my life are gone, and they all died in the house I live in. I nursed my husband for three years before he died of cancer. My mother died of lung cancer and my father died from a stroke. And I took care of all of them.

I don't know what it means to live this long. Recently, I began to worry whether Marilyn would be there for me if something happened.

I have always been the one who takes care of everyone. The thought never entered my mind that I could get sick or become an invalid. I have always been independent, and I was terrified of asking for help. I suppose I became afraid of every little thing that went wrong with me. I guess I got a little crazy calling Marilyn all the time.

The calls stopped after the third week of the sessions, and Marilyn decided to cancel the next visit to the social worker. Mrs. Marcus was a little disappointed, but she accepted what Marilyn had done. She was afraid of being a burden on her daughter.

Everything seemed to return to normal but not for long. The calls began again, and Marilyn scheduled another appointment. The session started with an angry confrontation when Mrs. Marcus accused Marilyn of being too busy to spend time with her. Marilyn and the social worker agreed to meet separately to talk about these feelings, but Marilyn was so upset after the session that she flagged a taxi for her mother and walked for several hours instead of returning to work. She wanted her mother to be comfortable and happy, but she was confused and frustrated. In her private session with the social worker, Marilyn talked openly:

> My mother has never been what you would call a happy person. But I want her old age to be happy. I have tried my best, but I just can't seem to make her happy.
>
> Before her operation she enjoyed spending time with the kids or shopping and cooking with me. Now all she does is complain that we don't spend enough time together. But that's not true. It is impossible to please her. When we're apart she calls constantly, and when we have time together, she complains or criticizes me.
>
> Last weekend, Mom and I sat in the backyard while my son and daughter played with friends. Mom told me that the children were scrawny and needed to eat more. Somehow it seemed like an accusation that I didn't care enough for my own kids. She made me so angry that I wanted to scream.

The social worker requested several more meetings with Marilyn and her mother. Marilyn agreed, although she did not believe her mother had the insight to benefit from counseling:

> Mom isn't the kind of person who will benefit from talking. She will insist the problem is mine, not hers.
>
> She'll say she is fine, and in the next breath she will sound weak and tell me I should make more time for her before she dies.

She sets up this double bind. It's exasperating to deal with her.

The social worker told Marilyn that things were not as mixed up as they seemed:

> Your mother understands that she is not doing well. She is terrified that something will happen to her, and she is even more terrified that you—who have always been there—will be too busy when she needs you! The surgery was the first time your mother had to confront a major personal problem, and it was a shock to her.
>
> She is not only afraid of growing old and sick. The toughest part for your mother will be to find the courage to ask for help when she needs it. Her endless phone calls are a way of acting out her fears. She wants to reach out to you, but she doesn't know how to do it! And I'm not sure you know how to reach out to her to deal with her feelings!

Both mother and daughter in this story were denying what was happening to them. Mrs. Marcus could not face an uncertain future filled with illness and losses. It was painful for her to face living and just as painful to consider dying. She was terrified of living because no one in her family had survived for so long. She was just as afraid of dependency and dying because she remembered vividly how her own parents and husband had deteriorated and died. Unable to face what was ahead of her and work through it, Mrs. Marcus developed physical and emotional symptoms of her fears.

The daughter too had her own denial system. Marilyn did not see that her mother was terribly afraid of growing old and sick. In Marilyn's eyes her mother was ageless. It was unthinkable that her mother, who was so strong and active, could get sick, need help, or die! Therefore, Marilyn blamed her mother for willfully manipulating her. Furthermore, she was consumed with the intense demands of her own career, and she did not want to deal with the consequences of a dependent mother.

Marilyn's denial effectively suppressed the conflict that might have occurred if she had confronted her mother's problem. Marilyn was preoccupied with legitimate responsibilities in her own world, but to confront her mother's dependency and fears would have created a situation for which she was not prepared. She sensed her mother's needs, but openly recognizing the situation would necessitate actions that were difficult for her to contemplate.

The dynamics of denial are "It's too upsetting to deal with," or "If I don't see it, it doesn't have to exist as a problem." Unfortunately, these dynamics constitute a barrier against analyzing the situation and developing strategies to respond to it. Marilyn and her mother's story illustrates what happens when aging parents and adult children cannot confront changes in later life. Most of us do not want to acknowledge our fears of change, whether we are growing up, growing apart, or growing old.

Marilyn and her mother needed help. Although help does not always mean a therapist, in this situation it is likely that the conflict would have escalated without professional help. Both mother and daughter might have become highly distressed, further prohibiting effective communication. It is even possible that Mrs. Marcus's problems would have taken the form of more "medical" concerns in an effort to get attention. Overt hostility or depression over perceived neglect might also have developed. Negative outcomes appearing as health-related problems can be the result of poor coping with stress.

Denial as a Natural Response

Confronting change is difficult at any age, and neither Marilyn nor her mother was coping with it well. Although aging parents and adult children experience life events differently, the specter of dependency and death is terrifying for both. If parents and adult children cannot face the fact that their lives have changed in a significant way, serious problems can emerge. Confronting the problems and sorrows that accompany a long life is often painful, but as hard as it may be to accept losses, illness, dependency, or just growing older, this realization is the necessary first step to overcoming denial. It is not unusual, however, for older people and their caregivers to engage in denial, refusing to acknowledge frailty, disability, and the need for help.

Older persons are less concerned about death than younger persons, but they are more afraid of dependency and disability. Still, death, especially sudden death, can be a painful shock to friends and relatives at any age. The tragic, accidental death of Bertha and Art Johnson and their children, a family who had been very close to Mrs. Marcus, had a profound impact on her and contributed heavily to her emotional distress. And it took several sessions before Mrs. Marcus finally confided in the social worker:

> Something awful happened the Sunday I returned to church following my operation. At the end of services our pastor announced that Art and Bertha and their two children had been killed in a car accident. Instead of filing out to shake the minister's hand, there was a rush to leave.
>
> I wanted to run, but there was no place to go. I needed to hide from the sick feeling inside me. I walked out of church stunned. . . . I even wanted to tell our pastor he must be wrong, that they couldn't be dead. The Johnsons were supposed to come to my house that afternoon.
>
> I remember trying to call Marilyn as soon as I got home, but there was no answer. I was angry and kept dialing over and over for what seemed like hours.
>
> When Marilyn finally answered that night, I must have been incoherent. It was like a bad dream. I thought I would wake up and everything would be the same again.

The reaction to the news of the Johnsons' fatal accident was key to understanding Mrs. Marcus's constant phone calls. Unexpected death is a shock to survivors who do not have the opportunity to prepare for death. For Mrs. Marcus, the sudden death of four people she had known very well, coupled with her deep anxiety about being sick and living alone, elicited such profound pain that she became ill in the aftermath.

If bereavement is prolonged, physical and emotional symptoms can emerge, and like Mrs. Marcus, such people will need help to overcome their pain. Her grief was so profound that Mrs. Marcus denied it and could not grieve. Her pain was too overwhelming and disorienting to her. Unable to express her grief and or deal with her fears, she resorted to the protective behavior of generating phone calls, which became so frequent that they alienated the very person to whom she was turning for support.

Unable to face her emotions, Mrs. Marcus turned her fear into the belief that she needed to hold on to Marilyn and keep her close. Unconsciously, she established the imperative: "Stay in touch with Marilyn so she will take care of me!" Mrs. Marcus was also afraid that Marilyn might be killed like Bertha and therefore taken away from her too! She called Marilyn constantly asking her to visit, because if Marilyn were with her, nothing could happen to her. Likewise, if Marilyn were always available, she would be there if Mrs. Marcus needed her. When Mrs. Marcus could not speak with her daughter, she panicked and the telephone calls escalated.

Therapy sessions for both daughter and mother gave them both greater insight into their impaired communication. Their relationship improved as Marilyn came to understand her mother's fears and need to be in close contact, and Mrs. Marcus recognized the inappropriate way she was handling her anxiety. Marilyn described her insights:

> I now know that Mom went "almost crazy" with grief and fear. I feel awful that I couldn't recognize what was going on then. I was so annoyed with her calls, her childish demands, and her criticism, it was all I could do to keep from screaming at her. I wanted to ignore her and stay as far away as possible. I guess she sensed this and that made matters worse.
>
> After the numbness left I felt overwhelming anger. I was angry with her for not telling me her real concerns. I was angry with Bertha for dying and angry with myself for being angry!

Unlike her mother, Marilyn had been able to grieve for the Johnson family. Allowing herself to deal with her anger and sadness was not easy, but the psychological pain gradually lessened as she allowed herself to think about the loss and to talk about it with others. In contrast, Mrs. Marcus had developed problems precisely because she clung to her denial.

The social worker helped Mrs. Marcus work through her denial by asking her to carry out several activities to deal with her pain. The first task was to visit the Johnson family grave with a tape recorder and some of her favorite mementos and photographs. Marilyn described what happened that day:

> Mom and I must have circled the cemetery at least ten times before we finally drove in and found a place to park. Neither one of us really wanted to do this. She thought it was silly, and the truth is both of us were upset, even a little scared. By the time we found their graves, I was in tears.
>
> I had to walk away to control myself, but Mom set things up. She had brought one of Bertha's scarfs and tied it around her stone. Mom unpacked two lawn chairs for us and sat with the tape recorder on her lap.
>
> She had written a series of letters to Bertha and taped them. I sat down next to Mom. She turned on the recorder and finally spoke: "Bertha, I want to tell you so many things. I wrote you a long letter and read it into this recorder. I wanted you to hear it—and I felt we should listen to it together. 'Dear Bertha, I want to say good-bye. . . .'"

Mrs. Marcus spoke later about what happened at the cemetery:

> My self-control was shattered when I said the words "good-bye," as I listened to the tapes and stared at the gravestone.
>
> I felt close to Bertha, and in that closeness, I felt my own dying. I knew that what happened to her could happen to me, and I felt cold dark fear.
>
> With the fear came anger, excruciating pain, a desire to scream at the wind, and a great heaviness. And I cried. I felt like a weight had been lifted from me.

Mrs. Marcus had begun the work of grieving. The encounter at the cemetery that had seemed so silly to her at first allowed Mrs. Marcus not only to cry but to cry with her daughter, for the first time. Driving home, they talked about many different issues. Both

Marilyn and Mrs. Marcus realized that they were survivors. They not only needed each other, they needed to evolve a new understanding about getting on with life.

Understanding Meaning in Later Life

Life review or reminiscence is a valuable strategy to work through withdrawal and denial. Mrs. Marcus began to heal herself when she was able to talk about death and feel it:

> Looking at Bertha's grave made me feel a mixture of emotions—pain, anger, sadness, and—it hurts to say this—happiness that I wasn't dead!
>
> I also felt guilty about feeling good that I was alive—a survivor. I knew I had to go on living, but I was afraid. What was I to do with myself? I was old . . . I had to go on, but for what?

During her next visit to the social worker, Mrs. Marcus began to examine what it meant to grow old. She was ready to discover herself and learn how to cope with the changes in her life. The social worker asked Mrs. Marcus to review important parts of her life. What were her earliest memories? What was she like as a young adult? How would she describe her marriage? Her job? What had it been like raising children? Who were the people who had affected her the most throughout her life?

The following dialogue shows how Mrs. Marcus saw herself. (The social worker's questions are italicized.)

What is the earliest memory you have?

I think I can remember being two—like the author Reynolds Price. He wrote about his earliest memory in a tribute to his parents. He was lying on a blanket and remembered the family pet goat trying to eat his diapers! My story doesn't have a goat! But I was in a tub of warm soapy water with our dog. Maybe it's not real. Perhaps it is a dream, but I remember Mom pulling me out of the water and hugging me.

Are you like your mother?

Oh, no! She was one of a kind. No one could be that loving and giving.

But isn't there anything about you that you share?

Well, maybe I'm a little like her. I try to help everyone.

Were you a good mother?

I hope so. I know I tried. Maybe you should ask Marilyn.

Do you feel differently about yourself now compared to earlier periods of your life?

Inside I am the same person. This body of mine is wrinkled and old, but the real me is the six-year-old child who loved going to school, the twenty-year-old who fell in love, and the thirty-year-old who quit teaching and cared for my family. I have devoted most of my life to my family.

What do you mean, you are the same person?

My home and my family were my world. . . . I've always felt that I had to do things for everybody to make them comfortable—my kids, my husband, my parents, my friends, even stray dogs and cats. Everyone needs someone to care for them, and I love taking care of things.

What has been the most difficult part of growing older?

Losing everyone . . . the pain of people getting sick and dying . . . not having anything to do . . . watching my body get old.

How do you feel now?

I feel empty. I don't feel seventy-nine. I don't feel any age. I am the same person I have always been. What is different is not having any meaning in my life.

Mrs. Marcus described herself as feeling "ageless." Despite obvious physical changes with advancing age, her perception of herself was constant. Sharon Kaufman has described this feeling of an ageless self as an almost universal perception. Mrs. Marcus had always had a clear sense of her identity as a giver, and most of what Mrs. Marcus talked about centered on her role as a mother and someone who gave care, not someone who received it.

Reflecting on the past, Mrs. Marcus said her mother was the most influential person in her life:

> I wish every person in the world could be as gentle and kind as my mother. Even as a young child I have vivid memories of how hard she worked. She took in laundry and did it all by hand. She mended clothes and made the most beautiful dresses from the material people brought her. She cooked and baked for our family and brought food to our closest neighbors who were very poor.
>
> Mother always made me feel safe and happy. She was always there for me. She loved being there for everyone!

"Being there" emerged as a powerful theme for Mrs. Marcus. As she talked it was clear that "connectedness" between mother and daughter and helping others had been driving forces in her life, but at age seventy-nine a major crisis loomed ahead—what to do for the rest of her life and what to do for others! Her oldest son was a prominent lawyer, and her youngest son a poor but happy actor in New York. Marilyn was successful in her business and a good mother. Bertha, Art, and the children were dead. No one needed her anymore and life was meaningless. What should she do?

The social worker proposed a way to find an answer to that question. She asked mother and daughter to participate in an exercise to help them understand how each perceived the world of the other. In this exercise, called "empty-chair interrogation," one person asks another a list of prepared questions, then answers the questions as if he or she were the other person.

The sample questions the social worker proposed for Marilyn to ask her mother were tough. When you were younger, did you have expectations about what growing old would be like? What is the hardest thing about growing older? The best? Do you think about the future? Do you have plans? What do you look forward to now? Marilyn resisted the exercise at first, insisting that her mother, not she, was the one with the problem and that besides, the exercise seemed silly:

> Aging is a nightmare to me. I see what has happened to Mom, and she is the strongest person I have ever known. If she's having problems, God help me when I grow old!
>
> I don't want to grow old. That's why I don't think I can do what you're asking. I don't want to know the answers.
>
> At the cemetery I saw death standing in front of me, and I knew Mom was going to die someday. That leaves me next. I don't want her to die and I don't want to die, but especially I don't want to grow old and feeble.

The social worker assured Marilyn that she understood what she was saying, but emphasized how important it was to participate. Her mother was on the road back to health, but she needed to communicate with the only person who could help her now—her daughter—and this exercise was a way to improve their communication. The social worker underscored that the mother-daughter bond was essential to promote better understanding for the two of them. The exercise might hurt, but after the hurt would come hope!

Marilyn finally agreed to participate in the empty-chair session. She sat facing an empty chair, with her mother and the social worker sitting behind her. She would read each question aloud, then answer it as she thought her mother would.

Q: When you married Dad, did you ever talk about what it would be like to grow old together?

A: Yes. We believed we were destined to love each other forever. We would grow old and gray, but that was unreal at the time. We had so much ahead of us. You were born a year later and then came your brothers, and so on.

Q: Aside from being with Dad, did you ever think about what it might be like to be seventy or eighty?

A: No. Looking back, I lived my life. We didn't have much, but we got along. I never wanted you kids to feel that you didn't have what you needed. I guess I was too busy trying to keep everybody happy and comfortable to think about being an old lady. Now I'm an old lady— with nothing to do.

Q: When you were fifty did you think about being an old lady?

A: Good grief, yes! That was a tough birthday. I was going through menopause and thought that life was ending for me. My clock had run out. I couldn't have more children, and you were all busy with your own lives. I didn't feel good about myself. I guess I saw growing old as going downhill to oblivion.

Q: What has been the toughest part of growing older?

A: Losing my role as mother—losing your father—losing my father and especially my mother.

Q: What has been the best thing about growing old?

A: I honestly don't know. I think it is probably living with my family. That's a hard question to answer. Right now, I don't see anything good about aging.

When Marilyn had finished with this sequence of questions and answers, it was her mother's turn. The social worker asked Mrs. Marcus to sit across from the empty chair. Mrs. Marcus was nervous as she began reading aloud the list of questions the social worker had made up for her to ask "Marilyn."

Q: How do you think you are like me?

A: I think we are too alike. Both of us are stubborn and determined to do things our own way. We find it easier to help others than to do for ourselves.

Q: How are you not like me?

A: That's a hard one. Perhaps the biggest difference between us is that I am more outgoing—more extroverted compared to you. I enjoy going out and being around different people.

Q: How do you think you are like your father?

A: I have Dad's temper and his need to attend to every detail. He always had to do everything a certain way. Every aspect of a meeting, trip, or project had to be carefully planned. I don't think I'm quite as bad.

Q: Do you think you will cope with later life better than I have so far?

A: I don't know. I just don't know, but I'm afraid.

Q: Can you picture yourself as a seventy- or eighty-year-old person?

A: No. I look at you and think that I might be like you, but I cannot imagine myself that old. I can't even see myself at age fifty. I'm not sure I want to.

Q: Have you thought about dying?

A: Yes, a great deal, especially since Bertha, Art, and the kids were killed. I've even thought about you dying. Someday it will happen—I don't want it to, but it will. I'm afraid of losing you.

Q: What will you do after I am dead?

A: I—I—I don't want to talk about your dying. It's too upsetting. I am not ready for you to die, but when it happens, I hope I can go on and make you proud of me. I will keep you alive inside me. You have given so much of yourself that . . .

Mrs. Marcus stopped the exercise when she saw her daughter in tears, and said:

Marilyn, you are in the prime of life, full of plans for your future. I only have a small amount of time left, but I can deal with my life again. You give meaning to my life and living, as well as my death and dying. I'm not ready to die, but I can look death in the face—and get on with living. I want you to see that too!

Mrs. Marcus and Marilyn continued their work with the social worker for several follow-up sessions to focus on plans for the future. Mrs. Marcus described it this way:

I never thought I would need help, but the counseling worked! My life and self-respect were like a shattered vase. The therapy helped me find each piece and decide what pattern I wanted to construct for myself.

Mrs. Marcus and her daughter found a new understanding of each other from this experience, including a shared realism about growing older. The experience of discovering each other's thoughts, expectations, and emotions had led not only to a fuller awareness of their relationship but to greater self-understanding and emotional independence.

The Emotions Behind the Problems

To confront denial means to feel, understand, and express the emotions behind the problem. Adult children and parents who overcome denial will be able to understand why each sees the world differently. Albert Schweitzer wrote that there is a "fellowship of those who bear the mark of pain." Those who are not part of this experience have a difficult time understanding what lies behind pain. To watch and care for a parent who is struggling with a chronic illness, without comprehending what lies behind their fear and pain, can be a barrier to identifying the scope of the problem as well as to understanding and dealing with emotions—theirs and yours.

For older parents, emotions may be responses to many different things and events that are happening to them. When older parents become ill, even when there are clear indications for recovery, their fears of getting worse, of not being able to carry out basic activities of daily living, and of needing personal assistance generate a great deal of anxiety and throw a dark shadow on the future. The prospect of losing control can become an overriding fear, changing the way they think about themselves. The anxiety and fear that accompany chronic illness become part of their identity.

Anger often accompanies illness, especially when pain is present. Among older parents it is common not only to become angry with family members but to be upset with them for not understanding what it means to be sick. Older persons are often subjected to many medical procedures, and in the process, they often become angry with doctors, nurses, and other professionals because they perceive them as indifferent or insensitive to their situation or because they have not cured them or cared enough!

Aging parents may also experience a wide range of emotions about having to sit or lie in bed while the rest of the world seems to be full of activity. Progressive loss of control and associated feelings of helplessness are common, and if they are not recognized and dealt with appropriately, they can lead to depression and "giving up" on life. Boredom is another common feeling; when coupled with helplessness and anger, it can lead to emotional paralysis—a lack of desire to set goals and try new activities, even when strength returns. Strange as it sounds, people learn to be bored, and this reinforces their underlying feelings that life is not worth living if there is nothing to do except experience pain and suffering. Isolation, fatigue, pain, depression, and boredom, in turn, all distort the thinking process, making it difficult for others to have rational conversations with people who are sick.

Sick people are caught in the dilemma of simultaneously wanting company and desiring to be alone. This dilemma often reflects the conflict between wanting independence and desiring help. Being alone conserves energy, which can be important when someone is very sick or in extreme pain. Trying to speak, move around, reach out for someone, or sustain a conversation can be painful and drain energy, but it is a way of fighting the terror of loneliness.

It is extremely common for older parents to complain vigorously that their children are not spending enough time with them. This complaint is particularly aggravating to the adult children who are actually devoting a great deal of time and making many sacrifices to help their parents. The parents' vigorous and often angry complaints are the result of a sick person's inability to deal with the dilemma of wanting both help and independence. Often the situation is further complicated by their inability to communicate what they really need or want. The overwhelming emotions associated with dependency often create powerful fears, and this too colors the ability to think clearly. Although adult children may reach out to help, their parents may not be able to "see" such overtures because their emotions blind them to what is happening.

Sometimes these conflicts are worsened when an adult child living hundreds or thousands of miles away makes a brief visit, hears a parent's complaint, accepts it as true, then accuses the sibling who has been providing most of the needed care of neglect and callousness to their parent. The caregiver-sibling who has visited the parent every day and fielded numerous emergencies, real and imagined, suddenly becomes the villain—victimized by a brother or sister whose personal involvement is limited to a weekly phone call, an occasional check, and flowers on Mother's Day or Father's Day.

Some older persons react differently to dependency. They pull away from family members in order not to be a burden and to protect themselves and their children from painful emotions and anxiety. But this behavior usually has the opposite effect—increasing isolation, disrupting honest discussions, and preventing mutual understanding—all of which are essential to knowing how to be helpful in restoring dignity and providing care with an acceptable quality of life.

There is perhaps no greater fear among older persons than that of long-term dependency. Most older individuals experience changes in their health and circumstances as very personal events, and they think about the future in terms of what their world is like and the resources that are available to them. For many, the desire for independence and mastery is powerful, and it is difficult if not impossible for them to adjust to an illness effectively and calmly. This is true at any stage of life, but in later life perceptions of self and emotional and physical strength may assume greater importance. This does not mean that older individuals always see themselves in the context of age. They deal with problems, changes, and disabilities as they arise, just as they have done throughout their lives. But they interpret these problems and changes in the context of what has happened to them in the past. What is important for adult children to understand is how a health "catastrophe" fits with older parents' perceptions of themselves and their ability or inability to manage.

Requiring others to help with personal needs generates strong feelings. Having to rely on someone else for help with dressing, washing, and toileting brings embarrassment and often a kind of despair that such easy activities are no longer within one's ability. Each such episode is a reminder of one's own helplessness and for many an embarrassment. These feelings, coupled with uncertainty about the future, in turn lead to anxiety, which family members see as chronic complaints and unpleasant encounters over trivial events.

Simply observing and experiencing disabilities and changes in your body or mind is distressing and lowers your self-esteem. It is difficult to feel good when your body is discolored, distended, unresponsive, or uncomfortable. Feeling bad about your body often engenders the paradoxical thought that the problem or illness is your fault, that you have failed in some way, that you could have done something to prevent those changes, or that you are inadequate, and that that is why you are sick or incapacitated.

Although there may be comfort in knowing that tests, procedures, drugs, and therapies may help, the feeling that you are not informed or involved in decision making can be a source of anxiety as well as hostility. When parents are so physically or mentally compromised that it is difficult to involve them in decision making, even the simple realization that they are not in control can be frustrating and upsetting to them. Resentment of people who give needles, take blood, administer drugs, or monitor vital signs is common. Hospitals, nursing homes, clinics, and other facilities can be seen as confusing, ritualistic, high-tech, hostile, and uncaring places, and tragically there may be more than a little accuracy in that perception.

Differences in perceptions about giving and receiving care are absolutely normal. Many parents' perceptions are not greatly different from those of hospital patients who believe they are being ignored by the nurses, even when nurses can document a high frequency of visits to these same patients. The message is simply this: Caregiving can yield a surprising lack of appreciation from a dependent, frail, and emotionally upset individual. This is often the end product of denial, anger that one needs such help, fear of dependency, guilt, and a desire to be rid of conditions causing the dependency.

Caring for the long haul depends on your ability to get beyond the momentary confrontations or carefrontations—and the associated impulse to leave or avoid such conflicts. Adult children need to deal with their own emotions maturely and understand and manage those of their parents—the subject of the next chapter.

3

MANAGING EMOTIONS

Effective caring is emotional business under the best of circumstance. It can be an emotional roller-coaster, in which positive emotions such as happiness, pride, and satisfaction are intermingled with negative emotions such as anger, fear, and sadness. Negative emotions are normal, but if they become persistent and overwhelming, they may undermine your ability to take care of yourself and your parents.

There will be times when you may feel overwhelmed by many different feelings, and there will be periods when you feel numb, washed out, or totally devoid of feelings. This numbness and inertia, along with the full potpourri of emotions, will cloud thinking, trigger arguments with others, and even make you feel that it is hopeless and impossible for you to do anything right. All of these emotions will diminish your effectiveness as a caregiver.

Since the stress of caring is so complex, it should not be surprising that you feel many different and upsetting emotions, including the following:

Anger and rage

Apathy and withdrawal

Anxiety

Depression or sadness

Embarrassment

Helplessness and hopelessness

Feelings of failure and inadequacy

Feelings of worthlessness

Frustration

Grief and despair

Guilt and shame

Panic

You may experience physical discomfort, for instance:

Sleeplessness or excessive sleeping

Stomach problems, or decreased or increased appetite

Skin rashes

Headaches, backaches, muscle problems

Rapid or pounding heartbeat

Chest pains or tightness

Sweaty palms

Teeth-grinding or jaw-clenching

Difficulty concentrating

You may also deny any feelings that your own body has a lot of aches and pains. Many people develop a wide variety of somatic problems and do not recognize that emotional reactions to distress often appear as bodily symptoms.

Finding constructive ways to manage your emotional responses is essential not only for thinking and acting effectively for your parents but for maintaining your own physical and mental health. Our own research, like that of others, has shown that as many as half of all caregivers develop serious health problems because of the stress of caregiving. This chapter describes positive strategies that you can develop to understand and manage your emotions, as well as tips to know when you may need professional help.

EMOTIONS ARE PART OF THINKING

Emotions play an important role in thinking. They undermine your attention, shifting your focus from what you are doing and onto the demand that the emotional experience creates. Most emotions are natural reactions that force people to deal with one set of concerns while they distract them from others. This shift may also create an emotional reaction in its own right. For example, if your concentration is disrupted because you are upset, you then become more upset because you cannot concentrate.

The following caregiving situations illustrate how emotions can come into play.

> Your father's morning appointment with his doctor ends with arrangements for admission to the hospital later that afternoon "to run some tests." You have to cancel an important business meeting that day to do this, but you cannot reach your clients to let them know.

> Your new boss requests that you meet in the afternoon to discuss the productivity of your division. You have just returned from a two-week leave that you spent with your sick mother. Your boss declines to give you further information until the meeting.

> Your ninety-year-old mother calls to tell you she has just had a car accident and is at the police station.

> You are packing to fly to your daughter's graduation from law school. She is first in her class and is giving one of the commencement speeches. Your father calls and wants you to rush right over because your mother is having another "attack."

Each of these situations is different, but all have something in common: They can be interpreted in different ways, and the interpretation that you construct will determine your emotional response. In the first situation you and your father may be relieved because the hospital tests will end your uncertainty about what is causing his symptoms; or both of you may be anxious about the tests because of the discomfort of the procedures and the possibility of a disturbing outcome. Your concerns about your father, coupled with the possible loss of a contract because of the canceled meeting, make you especially anxious. In the second situation, the meeting with your new supervisor could be good or bad. Your boss may feel that you have not been very productive and an unpleasant meeting may lie ahead. On the other hand, he may think that you have been doing a great job and want you to assume another big project.

In the third situation, your mother is shaken up, confused, and unsure about whether she will be found responsible and liable for damages. You are distressed and do not know whether the accident was serious or minor. You begin to doubt her ability to drive and fear the implications that having to drive her around in the future will have on your life.

In the fourth situation you may feel anger toward your parents for creating this dilemma. You wonder if the latest attack is a real problem or another histrionic effort to get your attention, knowing that you are leaving town. Since relations with your daughter have been strained in recent years, this trip has assumed great significance. You can ignore your father and take the flight, but what if something serious happens with your mother? Even if nothing happens, what will be your parents' reaction to ignoring their plea?

Your thinking about such events and the emotions surrounding them are the result of three ongoing processes. First, your mind identifies, incorporates, and interprets an event and then assigns meaning to it. Second, you immediately fill in any gaps in what you know with speculation and inference. And third, you actively search for more information.

The first process involves something called labeling—attaching meaning to the event. You interpret the need for hospital tests as meaning that your father has a serious health problem. You interpret your mother's accident to mean that she is no longer able to drive. You label your father's phone call as another overdramatization and manipulation on the part of your mother. The labeling process begins immediately, even before you have all the information necessary to make an accurate assessment. It also sets the stage for whether you will experience distress or a positive emotion with the events.

The second process occurs at the same time as labeling—you make inferences about the unknown, based on your attitudes and beliefs. You fill in some of the gaps in your knowledge with these inferences. What inferences you make are based on many different factors, including your personality, your view of other people, and the circumstances themselves. You may be pessimistic, for example, and the news that your boss wants to meet with you causes you to assume that your boss is unhappy about your work and may even fire you. Hearing of your mother's accident, you could assume that it was she who caused the accident because she had a minor fender-bender last month, when in fact she was the victim this time. When your mother calls you from the police station, you are sure she is acting out to get your attention.

Information-seeking is the third process. Acquiring new information is important, but it usually is something you cannot always get, and that may aggravate your emotional state. The doctor may not be able to disclose the test results for several days, which gives you more time to worry. Your boss may not want to discuss the meeting agenda, causing several hours of tense speculation. Your mother may be so shaken by the accident, even though she only sustained minor injuries, that she cannot give you a coherent story over the phone. You have to wait for the facts until you get to the police station. As you ask your dad for specific details about your mother's attack, he gets irritated and hangs up. You calculate the time you will need to detour to visit them on the way to the airport and still make your plane.

Therefore, the way you label events, your attitudes and beliefs about why things happen, and your ability to acquire information are all processes that depend on how your thoughts and emotions work together. Some emotions energize you to make decisions and solve problems easily, while others distract or prevent you from thinking and acting effectively. Furthermore, if you feel angry or anxious and are unable to find the information you need, you may feel still more anger and anxiety—which will keep you from looking for the information you need.

Sorting Out Feelings

Parents are emotionally powerful figures to their children, and when they need help, it causes many feelings to surface. Our beliefs about the love we did or did not receive from them as children, about how they treated us in relation to our brothers and sisters, the sacrifices they did or did not make for us, as well as our memories of countless critical incidents of our lives—all can affect our feelings as caregivers.

A lifetime of these experiences and feelings colors our thoughts and emotions. It is not unusual to confuse these charged memories of the past with our thoughts and feelings about our present circumstances. It would be strange if this were not the case! The purpose of caregiving is not to help us resolve a lifetime of feelings toward our parents and other relatives—this is impossible. What you need to do, rather, is sort out your emotions and understand how they may be helping you or hurting you, in order to manage them effectively.

When adult children are thrust into situations where their parents have legitimate expectations for assistance, the new dependency is jarring for everyone and elicits a range of emotions. The reactions of everyone involved to these dependency shifts sets in motion a series of events that can either strengthen or strain the family. If denial is the dominant long-term reaction of you or your parents, the process of healthy adaptation will be stalled. As we saw in the last chapter with Mrs. Marcus and her daughter Marilyn, denial can have severe consequences.

The key to beginning to cope with and manage emotions is to sort through the mess of your thoughts and emotions. *To sort* means exactly what it seems to mean. Many of us sort our emotions regularly, and some of us are better at it than others. Use the following list of emotional states as an exercise to help you sort out what is going on in your own heart and mind right now. Read the following statements, and check the ones that describe you now. This exercise takes some effort, but it can help you make your emotions concrete rather than let them remain as an abstract sense of upset and frustration. Knowing what your feelings are makes it easier to express them. This exercise can be valuable even if you are not in a distressing situation at the moment. Think about times you felt distressed by your parents, and go through the list below.

———— I feel lonely

———— I feel scared

———— I feel guilty

———— I feel embarrassed

———— I feel confused

———— I feel weak

———— I feel angry at others

———— I feel angry at myself

———— I feel frustrated

———— I feel sad

———— I feel useless

———— I feel powerless

———— I feel ugly

———— I feel anxious

———— I feel sorry for myself

———— I feel restless

———— I feel stupid

———— I feel depressed

———— I feel panic

———— I feel angry

After checking off your feelings, get a piece of paper and write several sentences about each emotion you selected. If you checked off "I feel anxious," for example, you might write:

I feel anxious whenever Mom calls me.

I feel anxious whenever I take her to the doctor.

I feel anxious when my husband criticizes me about being at my mother's house every day.

I feel anxious every time my boss calls me.

Clarifying the situations that provoke your emotional responses will move you from confusion to a more specific and concrete understanding of what aggravates or disturbs you. You can then begin to do something about your emotions. There are a number of things that you can do once you have identified your emotions. You can talk with someone to help sort out your feelings and thoughts, or just allow the feelings to be there, or find ways to work them out. Exercise, take time out for yourself, or do something for yourself. You can write about your emotions. Keeping a journal or diary is helpful, even with the most painful situations. A journal may also turn out to be useful to others who are trying to help you and your parents.

The story of Al Pruitt and his mother describes how one man used a diary as well as meetings with his family and nursing home staff to deal with one of the most painful decisions an adult child ever makes—placing a parent in a nursing home. Al began his diary one evening after a fight with his oldest daughter, who felt he was abandoning his mother by moving her into a nursing home. Al was unable to move around because he had sprained an ankle and broken a toe playing football that same morning. He was so upset by the argument that he needed to do something to defuse his anger. Since he was a newspaper columnist, he decided to write a story, pouring his thoughts and emotions onto the pages.

This led Al to begin a diary, which he kept the entire year his mother was sick. Recording his thoughts helped him come to grips with his personal anguish as he watched his mother deteriorate. The journal soon became a ritual without which he could not finish his day. Making daily entries became a way of anticipating the many tasks of caregiving and then developing a plan.

Keeping this diary has worked well . . . To make something of each day, even as Nana gets worse . . . a minimal goal, but more of a challenge than I ever imagined. Writing has been a form of therapy. I wonder how others escape the madness of this situation!

We take Mom to the nursing home today. I wish we could have waited a week or so, but I think we are all ready. . . . It's so gut-wrenching. It's her birthday.

Watching Nana wear down was tearing everyone in Al's family apart. Nana had lived with the Pruitts for eight years after her husband's death. Most of these years had been good ones. Al's mother had enjoyed her children, grandchildren, and greatgrandchildren, as well as done some substitute teaching. She was a talented amateur painter and writer, and she volunteered at the local elementary school until she broke her hip on an icy sidewalk. While she was recovering from hip replacement surgery, she suffered what appeared to be a stroke, which left her partially paralyzed. The decision to place Nana in a nursing home was a painful one, but after many family discussions it seemed the best, indeed, the only alternative.

The transition was easier than anyone had anticipated. After getting Nana settled, they celebrated her birthday, inviting the staff to share cake and coffee with them. After leaving his mother, Al asked for the first of several meetings with the staff. He wanted them to understand what his mother had been like throughout her life and, just as important, what it was like for her to be seriously ill—what she described as "on the down slope." He gave them his journal to read, brought in photograph albums, and told them stories about her. He created a real person for the staff to relate to, rather than an old lady who needed technical care.

EMOTIONS WHEN RELATIONSHIPS ARE NOT LOVING

Not everyone has tender and loving relationships with their parents and other family members. The reactions that occur when aging parents need help may trigger strong rejection, such as "They deserve what's happening to them," or "She never was there for me—why should I be there for her?" or "He's always been mean and selfish—even if I helped, he wouldn't appreciate it, so why bother?" Other responses may be, "I'll help, not because I like my father-in-law but because I love my wife," or "She at least deserves a decent nursing home—we'll get her settled and leave it at that."

In some instances a child loves one parent but rejects another, thereby creating a significant degree of tension and turmoil as loyalties and emotions become twisted and tangled. This is a later-life version of parent splitting.

Fred Andrews was a very successful corporate executive and was the subject of admiring articles in trade journals, where he was featured as one of the rising stars in his field. He was, however, an unhappy man who could not abide his father; at the same time, he loved and cared for his mother. To respond personally to the needs of his frail and chronically ill father was simply untenable for him. He rejected counseling as "unnecessary kid stuff" and maintained that since he was sending money to his mother, his father's care was taken care of. But then his mother became a problem. She was very upset and torn between her son and her husband. When Mr. Andrews asked, "Why doesn't Fred ever call? When he does call, you hang up before I ever talk with him," she could not tell him that Fred simply refused to talk with him. Fred's refusal to deal with his father was helpful to himself, but it was harmful to both his parents.

Recognizing and accepting any negative feelings we have about our parents is important before we can move on to make decisions about what we should or can do for them. The intent here is not to examine the limitations and failures of our parents' love; nor is it always possible to reconcile family responsibilities when relationships have become embittered. It may be understandable for some children not to feel obligated to their aging parents. Anger or contempt are tough encumbrances to carry, but these negative feelings are real and may be unresolvable.

You have at least three options in these situations: to ignore your parents' needs, to find someone else to help them, or to accept your emotions and do what must be done while retaining some emotional distance. When family relationships have been hostile or estranged, the demands of responding to chronic illness and death make caregiving difficult if not impossible. If bitter emotions exist, you should find someone else to help your parents if you have the resources. This deals with the humanity of the situation and gives you the necessary emotional distance. Neglecting parents in need, no matter how much you hate them, is a decision that you should carefully discuss with close friends, other family members, or clergy. Anger is a powerful emotion, but guilt over lost opportunities to reconnect with parents before death can be painful to live with the rest of your life.

Gianna Riccardo had been abandoned by both of her parents. Her father had left her mother when Gianna was only three, and her mother had placed her in a boarding school when she was eight, remarried, and moved away. Gianna remembered her mother and stepfather visiting twice after that, once when she was hospitalized with pneumonia at ten and the doctors thought she would die; the second was to arrange for her to study abroad. Apart from a few brief Christmas visits over the years the last time Gianna saw her mother was at her funeral. She recalls:

> I am glad Mother died quickly. I don't think I could have gone through the business of having to take care of her. She was my mother, but she wasn't really a mother.
>
> I have had a life without a father or mother. . . . It's sad, but being abandoned has tortured me as along as I can remember. I used to have this great desire to get revenge, but no more.
>
> There are still scars, but I have learned not to pick at them and leave them alone.

Although Gianna never had to do her own parent caring, she recognized the impact of parental neglect and talked about it with her husband. If your significant relationships have been negative and if your parents are in need, it is essential for you to find someone you trust to help you figure out the proper response.

Loyalty as a Powerful Family Emotion

Caring for aging parents creates opportunities for adult children to express loyalty or disloyalty. Children can repay their gratitude by being kind, loving, and supportive to their parents for the love they invested in them. On the other hand, aging parents are also an opportunity for "revenge" or settling the score for years of unjust treatment or neglect. In the latter situations, the payment is usually neither clear nor direct. A passive-aggressive person may find some presumably valid excuses not to fulfill commitments, thereby relieving his or her guilt but managing to express his or her anger. A rejected child can act out by rejecting his or her own family, then go to great lengths to care for a father or mother who was always aloof or distant. These behaviors may seem paradoxical, but they are attempts to compensate for years of unspoken anger and subsequent guilt as old, hateful wishes come true.

Loyalty is an important concept in caring. The family therapist Ivan Borzynmenyi-Nagy has described loyalty as the "invisible but strong fibers" that hold family members together. Loyalty is more than a feeling of emotional attachment between individuals. The French word *loi*, related to our word *loyalty*, means "law," and loyalty implies law-abiding actions and beliefs about "doing the right thing." What happens in family life over the years reflects the abilities of everyone to balance the loyalties that bind one another. Living together and sharing family events—marriage, divorce, birth, a new job, retirement, sickness, an accident—forges a rich bond of emotions and memories that outsiders can recognize but never fully share. Each generation and each family develops its own fabric of experiences, and this history, which exists in memory and emotions, is unique to the family members.

In many families the authority for decision making is clearly defined and rests with a parent or parents. Discussion is usually limited to advice seeking or unsolicited giving, but there is little consensus building in making decisions. In such families, what often happens is that as parents (and children) age, conflict or confusion about responsibility and authority begins to emerge. When the key decision-maker becomes impaired, the ambiguity increases and the dynamics of the family play a powerful role in the new family balance. Caregivers are often caught up in this process just when their energies are needed to deal with the challenges of providing care.

Every family develops its unspoken rules by which family members relate to one another and show loyalty. Some families are intimate, and individual members are deeply involved with one another. Others are congenial, but members spend less time directly involved with one another. In still other families members are indifferent to one another, and some families are angry and combative. Family loyalties are expressed differently in each of these groupings, and therefore there are no easy or correct prescriptions for emotional well-being as families age and parents require assistance. The concept of family loyalty and the implicit notion that it should be possible to balance relationships between members may not be realistic in all families, particularly where hostility and destructive behaviors have been the norm.

As a family responds to one family member's needs or desires, they may not be meeting those of another family member who feels that his or her needs are more important. When this occurs, the emotional reactions that are likely to result need to be dealt with. Anticipate such problems, and think of appropriate reactions. Conflict can be a healthy way to come to a resolution, but only if there are rules. Sometimes referees need to be brought in to mediate such conflicts and to ensure fair fighting. Open discussions and arguments may clarify the value of one person's idea over another's or change both people's ideas slightly to meet changing circumstances. The secret is to allow feelings to occur without letting them get out of hand. When mild emotional reactions are bottled up and not expressed, they merely become the fuel for a later time when a seemingly minor issue seems to break the dam and a torrent of overcontrolled, previously unexpressed feelings cascade over everyone involved. This is the sort of emotional outburst to be prevented by not allowing the minor problems to build up to an uncontrollable level.

How Guilt Comes from Family Life

The ways adult children respond to aging parents seems to depend, at least to some extent, upon an unrecorded family ledger of loyal and disloyal actions built up over time. This metaphorical ledger reflects a process of invisible bookkeeping that is seldom discussed—it deals with the exchange of love and support as well as goods and services over the years. The ledger is not a simple scorecard on which gifts given, time invested, rewards or punishments meted out, are recorded. Human actions are not easy to tally, but we all retain memories of who did what, when, and for whom, and this affects the way we behave toward one another. Particularly important, these memories are laced with emotions, so that the family ledger is a lattice of actions and feelings from shared experiences over time.

In general, families develop a complex bookkeeping system in the way each member relates to one another. Bridges of trust and commitment are established when people are available, responsive, or helpful to others; while distrust develops when they are unavailable, unresponsive, or hurtful. The ledger is usually not explicit because it develops slowly, with the complex and rich fabric of family life. Al Pruitt described his family ledger, using the memories of his parents and grandparents, as follows:

> It's hard to describe the intense bonds in our family. I have so many memories which together tell a story about a special kind of law and order in our family. Mom and Dad believed that family always had to be there for each other.
>
> Once as a very young boy I remember taking a walk with Dad right after Grandpa died. He held my hand tightly and walked very fast. At times he was almost dragging me along with him. We didn't talk—he just wanted me there.
>
> When I saw he was crying, he picked me up and began to walk very fast, knowing I could not keep up. He just held me in his arms until we reached the end of the block. He put me down still in a half-hug and looked straight into my eyes . . . "I miss my father. He was always there when I needed him, and now he's gone. You and I are the ones who have to look after each other."

The ledger metaphor is especially useful when trying to understand guilt. One of the toughest emotions to conquer, guilt is the feeling that we have not met the obligations that we perceive we owe to our parents. Even in the most loving and giving parent-child relationships, it is common for the child to feel that he or she is not doing enough, a belief that is often unjustified.

Guilt often gets in the way of effective communication with and management of sick parents, because adult children are inclined to expect too little from their parents and too much from themselves. There are many real reasons for adult children to feel guilty toward aging parents—and vice versa. Over a lifetime, it is hard to imagine that all expectations were always met by both parents and children. There are obvious situations where this is impossible: a son or daughter who has not visited often enough over the years or who has been absent from important family events because of work obligations. Likewise, adult children may feel that a parent neglected them during their childhood due to work or other commitments. There is probably not one of us who has never experienced guilt because we failed to meet certain obligations and responsibilities. Furthermore, almost every family has had serious disruptions in its history, where people said and did things they wished they could retract, even years later.

Regardless of what causes guilt, the challenge remains to get beyond it! First, you must acknowledge that there are a lot of things in the past that have transpired between you, your parents, and others in the family. Understand how your guilt feelings are affecting your decisions about your parent, before you make them. If you get trapped in a lifetime of guilt, you are doomed to be miserable no matter what you do. In addition, you may end up committing resources to your parent beyond your means—in the process sacrificing others who depend on you and ultimately depriving them of necessary resources, thereby setting up conflicts.

Although you may initially feel a sense of well-being in making good on your perceived debt to your parents, as time goes by, it will become obvious that you can never do enough, and feelings may sour. Likely you will begin to feel exhausted, hopeless, and resentful. This is precisely what happens after a lifetime of unchecked guilt: The guilt drives you to feel too ashamed to do anything except try to make up for all your perceived wrongdoings. You become like a caged animal running on an exercise wheel, getting exhausted but going nowhere.

Even when parent-child relationships are estranged or disrupted, guilt often surfaces to play a role in caregiving. It is legitimate to question your feelings of obligation to provide sustained care for your parents. Many adult children who have been abused and neglected by their parents nonetheless feel a sense of moral obligation to provide care for them. At the same time they desire to stay away. This is a natural bind, and the message here is not to neglect your parent but to recognize that a minimum response from you is acceptable. There is no formula for determining how much care is sufficient. In fact, this is the heart of the problem. Your feelings can lead you astray, and yet there is no meter that tells you that you are doing too much or too little.

Our suggestion is that by dealing with yourself and others openly, by bringing in others, and by listening, you can get some insight into what you are doing. It is up to you to figure out the "why." We are not suggesting that dealing with your guilt feelings is easy. The important lesson is to try to address and place the past and your feelings about the past into perspective and deal with specific tasks that will lead to a responsible level of care for your parents' well-being. You and others in your family need to focus on present tasks necessary to enable your parents to function at the highest level, consistent with available resources.

Our society lacks a cultural experience in which people live together as families for a long time. This fuels the guilt that many of us feel over the adequacy of our responses to our older parents. The rapid aging of our society is a historically unprecedented event, and we have not yet learned how to deal with our oldest generations. It has been suggested that we pay our debts to our parents by providing for their grandchildren, thereby continuing their heritage. While this may be the case in some families, not everyone has children. Furthermore, however much we care for our own children, it is a rare situation where we can ignore the needs of parents.

Our society does not yet give us a sense of how much we need to do to fulfill our obligations to our parents and still nourish ourselves and others. In the past, the ledger was balanced when each generation gave to the next the skills and resources it needed to survive. Parents died relatively young, and children invested in their own families without having to worry about parents. Today adult children must come to grips with what they can realistically do for their aging parents. The needs of a sick parent can seem virtually limitless and impossible to fulfill. This is true for any sick human being, not only aging disabled parents. Understanding that you may not be able to meet all of the needs of your ailing parent, however, is the first step toward untangling the Gordian knot of endless unmet needs and endless guilt. You can get into trouble if you do not set limits.

Carla Riviera described what happened when her sister Alice could not deal with her guilt when their father went into a nursing home.

> Alice visited Dad every day, sometimes twice a day for eight months. She fed and dressed him every morning. Dad sobbed and clutched her tightly whenever she tried to leave him, and it broke Alice's heart. As a result she would stay on most of the morning, unable to leave him. It finally cost her her job. At first her employer was supportive and even suggested job-sharing. Alice refused, insistent that she could manage.
>
> She often got angry with Mom for not being there enough and blamed her for Dad's problems. It was not unusual for them to have terrible fights. Sometimes they would go a week without talking to each other.
>
> Alice started drinking heavily after losing her job, which only made the conflicts with Mom more violent. With help from one of the nurses we finally persuaded Alice to get professional help. Eventually she got better and understood how she had lost control of her life.
>
> Dad died when Alice was in the hospital. To this day she still feels guilty for not handling things better and for not being there when Dad died.

Alice Riviera is not unusual. She wanted her father "to be loved until he died," but she could not set limits on what she should do for him as a loving daughter. The issue was not her devotion; family members often feel compelled to spend long hours in the nursing home, and for many people this is what is right for their family. Alice, unfortunately, ignored other parts of her life and soon became so overwhelmed that she could not make reasonable decisions. Although her employer was willing to be flexible at first, Alice's anger rendered her incapable of rational decision making. When she was asked to take a leave of absence, she became so angry that she quit! Not only did she lose her job, but she alienated her family and the nursing home staff with her constant, belligerent demands.

Her sister Carla reported that the anger Alice felt toward her family and the nursing home interfered with her ability to help her father.

> Alice said that she was the only one who really wanted to help Dad, and she berated all of us for not caring. However, the nurses told us that she had no patience with Dad and would yell at him and even strike him if he didn't mind her.
>
> Fortunately, one of the nurses convinced Alice that she needed help. I don't think anyone in the family could have convinced her. It took an outsider to break my sister's anguish, guilt, and anger.

FIND SUPPORT TO MANAGE YOUR EMOTIONS

Exploring our feelings is not easy, especially feelings toward a parent, spouse, or child. It takes time and effort and often courage to look at yourself, open to the possibility that your emotions may be the ones that are causing difficulties. Although you may feel pressured to make decisions rapidly, this is a false pressure. Very few of the problems you face require rapid answers, but the emotions surrounding the pressures create the pressure for immediate decisions.

The best decisions are usually made when you and your family make the time to examine the alternatives. Find time during the day to talk with your family and others about your feelings. Unfortunately, most of us work at solving personal and family problems when our energy is low—at the beginning or the end of the day.

Even if you have a strong constitution, it is healthy for you and your family to find help in managing the emotional components of caregiving. It is not a sign of weakness to talk about your thoughts and feelings with someone else. Quite the contrary: It is the mark of a healthy and successful individual. Most successful people have advisers. Indeed, the most successful leaders in business, government, law, science, and any other profession have many people around them to provide accurate and helpful advice and information.

Even if you have always considered yourself a private person or someone "who can handle things," you should not handle parent-caring alone, in most cases. Some rare human beings are effective by themselves, and if you are one who can do what needs to be done and manage your emotions, more power to you! But it is no disgrace to be among the more than 99 percent of the rest of us who need people to support them.

To be human is to feel emotions and even sometimes to have emotional problems. You can deal with your emotions by yourself or talk with your family, friends, or clergy. You can also get professional help in overcoming your emotional problems before they get worse. It makes good sense to get help before emotional dilemmas get so difficult that they interfere with your ability to get things done, or that they make you sick. Deciding to get help is a sign of wisdom and maturity. You are showing that you are strong enough to reach out to others and that you believe in your potential for overcoming your difficulty.

Help is available for most of us. Your family physician can treat you in the office or refer you to another professional, depending upon the severity of your emotional problem. Other professionals are trained to help. These include psychiatrists, psychologists, and social workers, as well as psychiatric nurses, marriage and family counselors, and therapists, as well as pastoral counselors. Mental health centers in the community are listed in the yellow pages. State and local professional societies as well as local mental health associations are excellent sources of referral for aid and advice. If cost is a problem, these groups can help you find care based on your ability to pay. Prompt and correct intervention can help most people return to a normal life. The stresses and tensions of caregiving may be eliminated, but you can learn to cope with them better.

The rest of this chapter describes the emotional problems that are most commonly reported by caregivers—depression, anxiety, and anger. We also provide checklists and self-rating questionnaires to help you determine how depressed, anxious, or angry you are. None of these tests is a diagnostic instrument for mental illness. They are merely screening tools to help you identify the level of distress you may be feeling and to highlight the need for help.

DEPRESSION

Every one of us has felt sad at some time in our life. Although sadness, also called depression, is unpleasant, it is a normal reaction to failure, loss, and bad times. Some people rarely report depression except when dramatic life crises hurt them. Most people experience a state of depression whenever failures, losses, and barriers threaten them in everyday life. Unfortunately, a small group of people are always depressed and live in a state of joyless oblivion.

The Many Faces of Depression

Depression takes several forms. In the first of these, a normal reaction to loss takes the form of depression or sadness; this is the form we all know well. People we love reject us, get sick, or die. We lose our job or do not get the job we want. Our children have problems with school, friends, alcohol, or drugs. Negative feelings are the normal reactions of human beings who are experiencing emotional pain.

When upsetting situations occur, we may react with sadness and feel helpless, empty, sad, and blue, or just flat and uncaring. We may lose interest in things around us and have trouble concentrating. We eat a lot, or we lose interest in food. At night we toss and turn and wake up in the very early hours of the morning, unable to get back to sleep. But after a short while, a few days or a week or so, we normally begin to feel better. Our problems may or may not go away, but we find ways to accept or deal with our losses, failures, and problems.

Depression can also be a class of serious illnesses that have a powerful negative impact on a person's life. Prolonged depression is a serious problem. Persistent feelings of worthlessness and isolation can lead to drug or alcohol abuse and suicide. There are several types of depressive disorders, the more severe of which include unipolar and bipolar depression. The hallmark of bipolar depression is mania—the occurrence at some point in a person's history of symptoms that seem the opposite of depression, such as an outpouring of speech, hyperactivity, a belief in one's ability to do great and important things, reckless spending, and the inability to sleep. Since bipolar depression always involves episodes of both depressive and manic behavior, in the past it was called manic-depressive disorder.

Unipolar depression is a serious illness characterized by persistent sadness and negative changes in mood and feeling, as well as altered patterns of eating and sleeping, weight loss, and a declining interest in sex and other pleasurable activities. It is often seen as a state of apathy or "the blahs," where there is no enjoyment in life and the future looks bleak, and feelings of hopelessness and helplessness are with you most of the time, as are feelings of failure and guilt. Depressed people usually have a strong impact on others around them, making others feel very sad or a bit angry just from being in their presence. Some are irritable and anxious, fidgety and fussy, and chronic nay-sayers—just difficult to be around.

Depressed people are often mistaken for having physical illnesses, since depressive states seem to be associated with increased sensitivity to pain, lethargy, and malaise. When depression occurs it will make anyone who is already suffering from a chronic illness feel worse. Behaviorally, most depressed persons simply care less for themselves, ignore good health care, fail to take medication, and generally appear to deteriorate. It is not unusual for other people to mistakenly believe that depressed patients are suffering from Alzheimer's disease or related dementias.

A major depression differs from normal states of sadness in

many ways—in the number of symptoms, how severe they are, and how long they last. Major depressive disorders are not just mood changes; they are truly incapacitating, and they affect a person's thoughts, behavior, and physical state. Because depressed patients often feel like failures, many of them feel that they are unworthy of help, and they may be hopeless about their condition to the point of not wanting to get help from a professional or the family. To be clinically depressed is to have an illness and need treatment. Fortunately, most people with unipolar depression can be treated effectively with medications, known as antidepressants, and with psychotherapy—preferably with both. Those with bipolar depression also have a good prognosis with treatment, usually with a drug called lithium carbonate.

The Signs of Depression

If you think that you or someone around you may be getting seriously depressed, there are at least four areas where you should be alert for symptoms. Look for changes in thinking, mood, behavior, and body functions.

Thinking. When you are depressed, you have a bleak view of yourself, the world, and your future. The easiest tasks seem insurmountable. You believe that everything you do is worthless or inadequate. Even when others judge your accomplishments as successful, you see your achievements as failures. Your style of thinking is pessimistic. You see your life as one bad event after another, with little prospect for change.

Mood. You may cry a lot, often apparently for little or no reason, or you may feel that you are beyond tears. You may feel overwhelmed with despair, apathetic, and filled with indescribable pain and hurt. You may feel tense, angry, and irritable. These negative moods are not constant; in fact, they usually vary depending on the time of day. Early morning is usually the low point. You want to stay in bed and sleep rather than face the day. If you get up and get going, your mood typically improves as the day goes on. Evenings are usually the best, although you may feel slightly worse in the late afternoon.

Behavior. Your behavior is affected in several different ways. You may become restless, unable to sit still, pace a great deal, or flit from project to project unable to concentrate. Or you may move very slowly, withdraw from pleasurable activities, and stay in bed all day.

Body functions. The way your body functions changes. You may feel numerous aches and pains, lose your desire to eat and drink, or develop an increased appetite. Or you may toss and turn, unable to sleep at night. Waking up very early in the morning is very common. Your gastrointestinal system may either act up or slow down but this is not surprising since you have changed eating and drinking patterns.

If you sought help from a psychiatrist or psychologist, he or she would interview you and then attempt a diagnosis according to specific standards. To be diagnosed with a major depression disorder using current diagnostic criteria, you must display five of the following nine symptoms:

1. Depressed mood

2. Loss of interest in usual activities

3. Loss of appetite with associated weight loss, or overeating with sudden weight gain

4. Insomnia

5. Slowed thoughts or movement, or agitation

6. Loss of energy

7. Feelings of worthlessness and guilt

8. Decreased ability to concentrate and think

9. Suicidal thoughts or actions

This list of symptoms is intended not as a way for you to diagnose yourself but to give you a sense of the dimensions of depression, as well as the indications that a visit to a professional could be useful. Since depression is the most common illness affecting caregivers, we want to give you an opportunity to test yourself.

TEST YOUR DEPRESSION

Do you want to know how depressed you are? The following test, developed by Leonora Radloff at the National Institute of Mental Health, and known as the Center for Epidemiological Studies–Depression test, may be enlightening.

Select the answer that best describes your situation over the past week, and circle the corresponding number.

0 = Rarely or none of the time (less than 1 day)
1 = Some or a little of the time (1–2 days)
2 = Occasionally or a moderate amount of the time (3–4 days)
3 = Most or all of the time (5–7 days)

During the past week:

1. I was bothered by things that usually don't bother me.	0	1	2	3
2. I did not feel like eating; my appetite was poor.	0	1	2	3
3. I felt that I could not shake off the blues even with help from my family or friends.	0	1	2	3
4. I felt that I was not as good as other people.	0	1	2	3
5. I had trouble keeping my mind on what I was doing.	0	1	2	3
6. I felt depressed.	0	1	2	3
7. I felt that everything I did was an effort.	0	1	2	3
8. I felt hopeless about the future.	0	1	2	3
9. I thought my life had been a failure.	0	1	2	3
10. I felt fearful.	0	1	2	3
11. My sleep was restless.	0	1	2	3
12. I was unhappy.	0	1	2	3
13. I talked less than usual.	0	1	2	3
14. I felt lonely.	0	1	2	3
15. People were unfriendly.	0	1	2	3
16. I did not enjoy life.	0	1	2	3

17.	I had crying spells.	0	1	2	3
18.	I felt sad.	0	1	2	3
19.	I felt people disliked me.	0	1	2	3
20.	I could not get going.	0	1	2	3

To determine your score, add up the numbers you circled for each question or statement. Your total will be between 0 and 60. If you scored from 0 to 9, you are in a nondepressed range. You are also below the average score of adults in the United States. A score of 10 to 15 places you in the mildly depressed range, and a score of 16 to 24 in the moderately depressed range. If you scored over 24, you may be severely depressed.

While a high score on this questionnaire is not the same as a diagnosis of depression, if you did score high—or, regardless of your score, if you think that suicide may be the only way out of your current situation—do not hesitate to see a mental health professional as soon as possible. Help is available for you and for your situation.

If your score fell in the moderately depressed range, take the test again in two weeks. If you still score in that range, please make an appointment with a mental health professional.

Tips for Coping with Depression

These useful tips for coping with depression were developed by the American Cancer Society. They have widespread value for all persons in mild depressive states.

1. *Try not to focus on yourself too much.* The cycle of depression continues when people think and talk about themselves and their problems too much. Be aware of this focus on yourself. Do not brood and mope around.

2. *Try not to use words like* can't *and* shouldn't. Use words such as *can* and *want to.* Think in the positive: "I can do something. I will go out. I will call somebody." When people

are depressed, their tendency is to think negative thoughts.

3. *Get involved in a project.* If you are depressed, you need to find ways to get out of yourself. Being with children or other people, or reaching out to others by volunteering in some activity will help you get your mind off yourself.

4. *Learn to say no once in a while.* You may feel depressed because you feel so trapped by some of the demands of caregiving that you have lost control. But you can say no once in a while if you feel that unreasonable pressures are being put on you by others.

5. *Talk.* Keeping your feelings bottled up inside only increases your tension. Talking with someone may help you get a new perspective on yourself. Talking will also stop the cycle of introspection, brooding, and self-pity that is characteristic of depression.

6. *Know your limits and limitations.* You need to come to grips with what you can and cannot do. Know how much you can do before you get tired. Pace yourself.

7. *Rethink your need to win all the time.* There are many people who always need to be right and win every argument. Your depression may be caused by your need to be right when you are with your parents and other family members. When you do not win, you feel let down and rejected, which leads to anger and depression. Learn to give in once in a while.

8. *Exercise.* Physical activity is a great way to blow off steam and release your tension and frustration.

9. *Find activities that give you pleasure.* Spending time in a club or group or starting a new hobby can be therapeutic. Stop sitting around—get out and do things. Replace your feelings of sadness and self-pity with joy, happiness, and humor. See a funny movie, read the comics, and make it a point to laugh every day.

10. *Think about positive things.* Focus on what you have accomplished, not what you did not or could not do. Use your talents and skills, and think about your successes!

11. *Develop good nutritional habits, and get enough rest.* Depression can be caused by not eating properly or by not getting the rest you need. Don't eat alone. It's more fun to eat with others.

12. *Don't let life overwhelm you. Take one day at a time.* Figure out what is most important, and do it. If you let yourself be overwhelmed, you can become paralyzed and unable to function, which leads to depression. Write down what you think all of your problems are. Then look at the list and prioritize the problems. Choose the most important one, and list your options for dealing with it. Then devise your plan and list the steps to carry it out. Give yourself a deadline, and meet it!

These excellent tips can help you reorient minor depressive symptoms. If your depression is too disruptive, however, you simply may not be able to do what is needed, and certainly you should seek help in such cases.

Depression is a treatable state, and mental health professionals can make a difference. Not only are depressed people unable to act as effective caregivers, they themselves need help. In extreme cases suicide is associated with depression. Suicide can grow out of the intense feeling of helplessness and hopelessness often associated with guilt and/or anger, which are primary characteristics of the disorder.

In understanding depression it is worth noting that many physical illnesses (such as low thyroid activity) have depression as a symptom; that many medications (such as some for blood pressure control) may cause depression; and that depression, particularly bipolar depression, may have a genetic basis that increases an individual's vulnerability. Some depression is personality induced, and indeed some people have a chronic depressive mood for years.

Careful evaluation and treatment can lead to remarkable improvements in quality of life and under some circumstances to prevention.

ANXIETY

Anxiety is often a normal response and plays a helpful role in survival. Anxiety motivates us to avoid danger, take our children to the doctor when they run a high fever, install smoke detectors in our homes, run from burning buildings, and try to achieve better grades in school or focus in life. It is natural for people to worry, and this is a powerful motivation to make sure that we avoid danger.

People usually experience anxiety as a worried, uptight feeling. It can be a vague fear that something bad or unpleasant is going to happen to them, even when there is no threat. Anxiety may result when people hold back feelings they cannot cope with or do not understand. It may also grow out of a conflict between what they think they would like to do and what they think they ought to do.

The most common signs of anxiety are:

Nervousness

Trembling

Dizziness

Inability to slow down

Abnormal eating habits

Pounding heart

Sweaty palms

Nausea

Stomachache

Trouble breathing

Like many other conditions, anxiety may be helpful in small amounts and in specific instances. But in large doses it becomes a serious problem. So-called free-floating anxiety makes everything different and fearsome, and in the extreme, it is so overwhelming that it acts to prevent people from doing or trying anything. Anxiety can take other forms involving specific aspects of life. Overwhelming anxiety about appearance, for example, can lead to disorders where people literally starve themselves to death; fear of leaving home can become a phobia that prevents a person from working or going anywhere. Cleanliness can become an obsession, and hand-washing becomes the dominant activity of one's waking hours. Some people experience anxiety about many things and live with a pervasive sense of fear and dread.

There are many good reasons to feel anxiety about your parents' health or living situation. If your mother is being discharged from the hospital after a hip fracture, you may well worry about how you and other family members will be able to juggle work schedules to care for her as she recovers. If your father has a heart attack, the anxiety and fear can be intense until you know the outcome.

Remember that anxiety is a natural and helpful response to stress. It motivates you to do something. But prolonged, excessive anxiety can lead to serious problems such as ulcers, high blood pressure, psychiatric disorders, and an inability to enjoy life. Anxiety can also indicate an underlying depression. If anxiety interferes with your ability to function, it should be alleviated.

Symptoms of Anxiety

Anxiety can be overwhelming, make your life absolutely miserable, and interfere with effective caregiving. If you recognize yourself in any of the following three descriptions, you may want to consult a doctor for an evaluation. At the very least, talk with a friend if you are worried about yourself. Sometimes getting the support of someone you trust gives you the courage to visit a professional. Remember, your health is important, and all of these problems are treatable. It is not necessary for you to suffer!

Generalized anxiety disorder. This is characterized by constant, excessive, and unrealistic worrying, and often the following:

Restlessness

Tension and irritability

Keyed-up feeling

Difficulty concentrating

Sweating

Poor sleep

Lump in the throat

Dry mouth

Gastrointestinal disorders

Panic anxiety attacks. Severe, unexpected, intense anxiety attacks that occur without any apparent cause are known as panic attacks. They come on at any time, with no warning, and they seem uncontrollable. Someone in a panic attack is likely to experience the following:

Chest discomfort

Pounding heart

Shortness of breath

Smothered feeling

Fear of dying

Trembling

Light-headedness

Sense of losing control

Avoiding places where help might not be available if you need it

Obsessive-compulsive disorder. The anxiety disorder known as an obsessive-compulsive disorder is characterized by obsessions (the recurrence of intrusive ideas, impulses, or images) and compulsions (senseless, repetitive, and excessive behaviors). Usually, attempts to stop these behaviors lead to great anxiety.

Remember, these descriptions are not for self-diagnosis. They are meant solely to give you reference points to think about your level of stress.

Tips for Coping with Anxiety

Some tips for coping with depression apply to coping with anxiety. It may also be helpful to see your physician. A checkup is important if you are worried about your physical symptoms. Your physician will usually be able to diagnose the cause of your aches and pains. In the case of severe anxiety, panic attacks, or phobias, a referral to a mental health professional is also in order.

In their book *Anxiety Disorders and Phobias,* psychologists Aaron Beck and Gary Emery have suggested a five-step strategy to cope with anxiety. The trick to getting out of an anxiety state, they maintain, is to accept it. This may sound odd, but the following description clarifies the exercises you can learn to accept your anxiety. Using their strategy, you should be able to accept your anxiety and make it disappear.

1. *Accept the anxiety. Accept* is defined in the dictionary as "giving consent to receive." Agree to receive your anxiety.

   Do not fight the anxiety. By resisting, you are actually prolonging it. Try to replace your tension and anger with acceptance. Go with the flow.

2. *Watch your anxiety.* Look at your anxiety without judging it. You are not your anxiety. Be detached, and try to separate yourself from the experience. Rate your anxiety on a scale of 0 to 10, and watch it go up and down. Look at your anxiety as if you were an outside bystander.

3. *Act with the anxiety.* Act as if you are not anxious. Try to normalize your situation. Breathe deeply. Stay with your anxiety and function with it. Try not to let your mind run away with the overwhelming need to block off the upset.

4. *Repeat the steps.* Continue to accept your anxiety, watch it, and act with it until it goes down to a comfortable level. It will if you repeat these steps.

5. *Expect the best.* Try very hard to change your mind-set to expect the best. Think about good times in your past when you were happy, and remember the feeling. Use this technique to energize yourself to entertain the notion that good times may be ahead again.

What you fear the most rarely occurs. As long as you are alive, you will have some anxiety. Do not be surprised by it. Expect it, and expect that you will be able to handle it.

ANGER

Parent care can generate a lot of anger. Being on the front line with aging parents changes your life in many unanticipated and often undesirable ways, and it does not feel good. Anger is often a coverup for other emotions that are difficult to face, such as fear, guilt, helplessness, and hurt. If you are angry, it is likely that this is your way of dealing with one or more of these other emotions.

Anger can have strong negative effects on you and your family and friends, particularly if you are angry all the time and creating conflicts within yourself and with others. Your anger may show itself as jealousy toward others if you resent their good fortune or health. You may feel that nobody understands how uncomfortable or upset you are. People around you may seem insensitive, and you may think, "How dare the world go on as usual when I have such problems!"

You may look for someone to blame for what has happened to you or for your hurt and angry feelings. You want a target for your anger—the doctor who made you wait an hour for your appointment, the woman driving slowly in the car ahead of you, or your dog for needing to go outside to relieve himself at an inopportune time. You will also blame yourself: "How could I be so stupid! I should have done something sooner—I saw how Mom had been slipping, but I let it go on!" For religious people, God often receives blame: "How could God desert me when I need Him most?" or "What did I do to deserve this?"

Frustration over not being able to achieve your goals can be particularly anger-provoking. Wanting something in a particular way and at a particular time is setting yourself up to be frustrated, particularly if you do not take the wishes of others into consideration. Prevent yourself from entering this trap by maintaining a flexible and cooperative attitude (see Chapter 4).

Even people who are usually even-tempered or easygoing can develop a short fuse under the stresses of parent care. You may suddenly feel that the whole world is out to upset you. The simplest incident can trigger a massive anger response—a casual comment by a friend annoys you, the sandwich delivered for lunch is not the one you ordered, or the homeless man on the street asks you for money—and you curse him under your breath for being a drunk or too lazy to get a job. Anger is triggered by whatever happens to be in your way when the last emotional straw is laid on your back. The ostensible cause of the anger does not have to make sense, although you always seem to yourself to have good reason to be mad.

Anger can be an appropriate and sometimes helpful response, depending on the circumstances. Anger frequently begins to surface as you work through denial. As the shock of an event wears off, you may feel enraged: "It's not fair!" or "Why me?" are common thoughts. Even though the anger may not feel good, it catalyzes a healthy healing process because it gives an outlet for the upset, frustration, and helplessness that often occur throughout the course of parent care. Anger can be appropriate when the health professionals and others upon whom you rely are not helpful to you or your parents. Many professionals are not trained in geriatrics and may not always be able to tell you what you want to know.

Options for Expressing Anger

Exploding at the person or event that makes you angry will probably not be very effective. It may only make you more frustrated, create guilt over losing control, and lead to even stronger feelings of anger. It is important to find nondestructive ways to express your anger. Regina Sara Ryan has suggested several techniques in her book *The Fine Art of Recuperation.*

Work it off. Do anything that allows you to vent the feelings you do not know what to do with. Beat a sofa or bed. Throw a pillow. Give yourself permission to let go of the steam built up inside you.

Write a letter or draw a picture. Express your anger on paper. If you do not feel like writing, speak the letter out loud. If you are unable to compose a letter, just write words that represent your anger. When you are finished, destroy the letter or drawing: Mark it up, scribble all over it, or tear it into pieces.

Take a shower or bath. This is an easy way to change your environment. Wash the anger out of your system: as you soak and relax, or vigorously scrub, imagine that the tensions inside you are flowing out of your muscles into the water.

Exercise. Take a walk, go jogging or swimming, or go to a health club to work out your anger.

Express your anger with a friend. Find someone to let you act out or talk about your anger. But do not project your anger onto the person with whom you are talking.

It is normal to be angry and to express it. After you relieve your anger, call a friend, get a massage, go to a good movie, take a nap, or find something pleasurable to do.

When you can identify your emotions, give yourself permission to feel them, and understand why you experience them, you are in a position to function more effectively with other people in the tasks of caring. The next chapter describes how to build collaborative partnerships with others to do what you need to do.

4

BUILDING COLLABORATIVE PARTNERSHIPS

Caring for aging parents involves not only thinking and dealing with your emotions but taking actions. You will have a variety of tasks to carry out, and in most instances, you will do best with help from doctors and other professionals, as well as in working with your parents, other family members, and friends. Working with people requires people skills, and some of us have better ones than others. This chapter will help you think about your people skills as a caregiver and highlight some approaches that you should find valuable.

In some ways, helping older parents and dealing with your family are like running a family business. Tasks like managing the financial aspects of care, coordinating the people directly and indirectly involved, mobilizing technical and professional support, and finding housing and transportation are also tasks done by managers and executives in business. What does the business world tell us about a successful manager? What qualities make an effective person? If you are an effective person:

- *You know yourself.* You know why you do the things you do, and you understand what upsets you. You have the confidence to know what you want to do and how to do it.

- *You are aware of the impact you have on other people.* You understand who is afraid of you, who likes you, who is pleased to see you, and who resents your presence. You understand that your energy and influence attract some people and scare others away. You can sensitize yourself to establish collaborative working relationships to do the job that is needed.

- *You can accept weaknesses.* You know what you and others can and cannot do. You can get help to make up for your weaknesses and find others with the abilities or skills to help you.

- *You can identify strengths in others.* You can share responsibility with others who have the strengths and assets to get a job done. You can analyze the strong points of others and integrate them into your plan.

- *You can accept others who are different from you or who think differently from how you do.* You know how to get others who think and act differently from you to show their talents. Creative solutions to problems emerge because you are able to involve those who "march to a different drummer."

- *You have a flexible style.* You know that even when your plans are working, something unexpected can happen and you will need to change your course. You are able to "go with the flow" or "bend with the wind"—that is, you are prepared to change when you need to do so.

- *You create a trusting environment for people to think, work, and live in.* Trust is one of the most difficult virtues to cultivate in a group of people, but it is the glue for human relationships. You can build trust upon a record of your experience, so that people say to you, "You were there when I needed you and I will be there for you. I know you will follow through."

- *You can manage conflict.* Conflict can be a response to a complex situation where people see different possibilities and are acting on different information. You give people the opportunity to express their views and emotions and can navigate in rough waters.

If you recognize most of these characteristics in yourself, then you should have confidence that you are likely to be an effective caregiver. If you do not see these characteristics in yourself, there are several very important tasks for you to do. Think about the other members of your family, and identify who has these qualities. Make an effort to talk with that person and advise them that they are needed to exert leadership in the family. One of the greatest qualities of any human being is to recognize what you cannot do, then find someone to do what must done.

Building a Partnership with Your Parents

You do not have to be entirely devoted to your parents or even love them to care for them. When your relationship has been poor or estranged, it is legitimate for you not to spend a great deal of personal time with them or to get involved in mutual decision making. Where relationships with other family members have also been estranged, it is not necessary to reverse a lifetime pattern because your parents are sick. In some instances parental needs catalyze repairs in the family, and this may be desirable. The point, however, is that it is not necessary.

When your relationship with your parents has been good, reaching out to them when they need assistance may still feel awkward or uncomfortable. The shift in relationships and your acceptance of parent care is a new experience for everyone. It can be very helpful, particularly at the outset, to keep the issues on setting goals, developing plans, and determining who will be needed to help carry them out. The more focused you are, the easier it will be to discuss these issues.

One of the challenges of caring for aging parents is that they often need help getting assistance or services from a wide range of people and professionals—from physicians and other clinical specialists, to professionals in various community agencies, to lawyers, financial planners, and many others. There are three steps you should take before you make contact with any professional on your parents' behalf.

1. Talk with your parents about the importance of working together in a partnership of mutual responsibilities. They may be shy or afraid to ask for your assistance, so volunteer to be there for them. Let them know you are all in this together.

   Unless your parents are severely incapacitated, the decision-making authority resides with them. You may wish to advise and share the decision making, but as long as they are competent, that too is their choice. With their cooperation you should explore the likelihood that medical decisions will need to be made at a time when your parents are not able to make such a decision. A limited power of attorney agreement can be of great value to the family and can provide peace of mind for your parents and you. This document recognizes that care will be provided as your parents wish, preventing conflicts and confusion and expediting care. A detailed discussion of this issue and related concerns can be found in Chapter 7.

2. Develop a list of questions that you and your parents have about medical problems, medications, and other health problems, as well as legal, economic, and housing issues. List everything, no matter how silly or trivial it may sound to you.

3. Share the questions with other relevant family members and solicit their input. Invite them to meet with you and your parents to discuss the problem areas you have identified. Secrecy at this point could lead to suspiciousness and later allegations that you used untoward influence to achieve your personal aims.

What do you do if your parents hesitate or refuse to participate? How do you confront the real and terrifying concerns of parents who do not want to become a burden? How do you enlist help when you are ineffective? Although there are no absolutes, there are some helpful guidelines.

- *Be accepting of your parents, without attacking them or acting as if only you know what is best for them.* One of the toughest aspects of dealing with older parents is resisting an authoritarian "know-it-all" approach, especially if you have done some research on the problem and you feel you know the answers. Your insistence will usually just alienate them. Even if you have information or ideas and feel you are better informed than they are, resist your legitimate impatience to take action. Share the information you have gathered with them, and carefully listen to how they respond to you. Be sure to provide them with any written information you may have found and agree to explain things.

- *Focus on the consequences of their behavior and try to defuse your own anger or frustrations.* Emphasize how important it is for your parents to let a doctor know about their symptoms and do an examination. Remember that early detection prevents pain, illness, and suffering since treatment is usually easier and more effective in the early stages of an illness. If they delay seeing a doctor or getting necessary help, their health could get much worse. By the same token, seeing an attorney or an accountant early on may be necessary and prevent later grief. Your parents may indeed know that an ounce of prevention is worth more than a pound of cure—but acting on this is easier said than done at any age.

- *Look beyond "old age."* Do not let protests of "It's only old age!" keep you from getting help. Research has shown that a substantial number of older persons blame old age for medical conditions that in fact can often be cured or managed. Sadly, the "old age" argument is frequently used by many physicians who say, "What do you expect at your age?" This attitude is harmful to anyone's health and well-being!

- *If absolutely necessary, force a confrontation and start an argument.* Sometimes an argument is a legitimate way to clear the air for honest discussion, but be aware of what you are doing and do it carefully. Let your honest feelings be known, but do not lose control of either your temper or the situation. Try to listen carefully to your parent and hear not only their words but how they express their thoughts and feelings. It is also important, however, that they know how you and others feel about them and what their behavior is doing to the rest of the family.

- *Know when you may not be the most effective agent of change.* Sometimes it is necessary to surrender control to another person. This is not a defeat—it is good strategy. It may be easier for your parents to deal with another relative or with a friend or a minister. This is not just saving face; it may simply be that they are more comfortable talking to someone besides their own child. It is a sign of strength on your part to involve others appropriately to achieve the primary goal— helping your parents. Do not insist on being the heroine or hero. Remember that the goal is to get the job done. Credit for getting it done is of lesser consequence at this stage.

BUILDING PARTNERSHIPS WITH YOUR SIBLINGS

Working cooperatively with your brothers and sisters can make parent care a lot easier, at least when your relationships with them have been good. Most sibling relationships are positive by the time people mature into middle age. Studies suggest that 80 percent of people have good relationships with their siblings, while only 10 percent are apathetic and another 10 percent are hostile. It also appears that sister-sister and brother-sister pairs have better relationships in middle and late life than do brother-brother pairs.

However, parent-caring usually revives old roles of sibling rivalry, and patterns of competition for parental love and affection may reemerge. It is also likely that difficult problems will develop when brothers and sisters help parents. Although many brothers and sisters will be able to manage the challenges of collaborative care, old issues may surface. For example, who is going to call the shots? Who decides when Mom and Dad go into a nursing home? Why does big brother think he is the boss again? The task is to recognize the possibility that old patterns may reemerge and be ready to deal with them maturely and with good humor.

When relationships among brothers and sisters have been troublesome in the past, getting everyone to help with parent-caring can be a challenge. Examine the possibilities carefully before you start the process. There are several questions you should ask yourself: What are the behaviors of your family? Who is close to whom? Who is estranged? What do your brothers and sisters believe are their responsibilities for your parents? How constructive or destructive are your siblings—and their spouses?

Remember that even within one family there can be striking cultural differences. When families have immigrated from abroad, older children who were raised initially in the other culture may share the parental values, while younger siblings may have very different values and expectations. Value systems may also vary when siblings differ significantly in age or are the offspring of remarriage by one parent. Keep in mind, too, that when your siblings marry, they become part of an entirely new set of relationships that you share only tangentially.

The complexities of modern family life can challenge the efforts of siblings who are trying to pull together as a group. The strong positive bonds between brothers and sisters can be classified into three general categories: loyal, congenial, and intimate. In loyal bonds, the siblings will always be there for one another, even when they are not friends. The congenial bond is one where siblings may be close to one another but turn to other relationships in a crisis. Intimate relationships are those where siblings get support from each other that they do not get from others. As families age, the bonds between siblings can become more important in the caring process, but you should not assume that your brothers and sisters will always be available when you need them, as the following story illustrates.

José and Flor Garcia had moved to the United States when their two daughters, Maria and Lourdes, were ten and five years old, respectively. Life was difficult at first, but they worked hard to start a new life. The Garcias were especially proud when a third baby girl, Estelle, was born exactly three years from the date they arrived penniless in the United States.

The girls grew up speaking Spanish at home and English in

school. They all did well and married after they finished school. Maria, the oldest, lived closest to her parents. Her two sisters lived several hours away, but they still visited several times a month.

When Mrs. Garcia first developed high blood pressure, it was Maria who made sure that she had a good doctor and monitored her medication use. At the time of Mrs. Garcia's first stroke, all the daughters came to the hospital and they also helped their dad, then in his late seventies, through the first few months of his wife's recovery. Over the next two years Mrs. Garcia suffered several more mild strokes and had increasing problems with her memory. Finally, under pressure from Lourdes, who had become a pharmacist, Maria took her mother for an evaluation. There they learned that Mrs. Garcia had a moderate to severe dementia secondary to small strokes in her brain.

Mrs. Garcia slept relatively little at night and dozed during the day. When she was awake, however, she wandered around the house moaning and cursing. It got so bad that Mr. Garcia told Maria that he wanted to move into another apartment. In fact, one day he drove away and did not return for two days, leaving Mrs. Garcia alone.

Maria told her sisters that they would all have to take turns staying with their mother so that one of them would be with her at all times. This worked for a few weeks, but then Lourdes and Estelle began to challenge Maria. Maria's response was to get angry and move her mother into her own home. She called her two sisters each day to berate them for not caring about their mother. Both Lourdes and Estelle worked to find their mother a good nursing home, and they resented Maria's continuing demands that they take turns caring for their mother.

Maria found herself alone, separated from her mother by the dementia and from her sisters by their mutual anger. She vented her anger on the doctors at the clinic for not giving her mother more medication to "at least keep her knocked out and quiet." One day, after three months of this anguish, including the hiring of five replacement aides, Maria went to the clinic in desperation. It was only then that a meeting could be arranged with the three sisters to develop a shared strategy to mend the fractured family.

When there are other family members to help you, it is important for you to know how to involve them. Talk together about your resources, and involve everyone who is appropriate to plan what needs to be done. Calling the family to meet together can prevent much of the aggravation of "she said—he said" that has such a bad effect on communication.

At the meeting, describe what you see as the problem, and share your expectations with your siblings. Let them do the same. Do your siblings have other problems that are causing a pileup of life stressors? If other family members are sick, you may need to accommodate their needs—at least for a while.

At first you may find it difficult to reach out to your siblings. It may be easier for you to do it yourself. Indeed, many caregivers say that they would rather do everything themselves than involve other members of the family. But it is precisely this kind of thinking that can lead to serious trouble. Long-term caring can seem interminable, and the trick is to find the best way for everyone to work together as a team, including the person who is sick. How to do this is the focus of the next chapter. The rest of this chapter examines your relationships with professionals.

BUILDING PARTNERSHIPS WITH PROFESSIONALS

If you were establishing a business with several partners, all of whom were sharing the risks, responsibilities, and profits with you, you would no doubt be asking many questions of each other. The same principle holds when you are building partnerships with doctors, lawyers, and a wide range of professionals.

Talking with doctors and other health specialists, lawyers, police, and community agency personnel can be a frustrating and upsetting experience. Too many people are afraid to ask questions of those they perceive as authority figures. If you have not already discovered this, you will find that many professionals do not communicate effectively with their clients. Since understanding the problem and communicating with those in a position to help is so crucial, it is important that you develop a sense of confidence that you can negotiate respectfully and thoughtfully for the information and services you need.

We propose seven guidelines for you to consider in these situations.

1. *Let the professionals you are dealing with know that you and your parents or other family members are working together to deal with the problems you face.* Ensure that you are in a position to obtain confidential information, if necessary, by spoken or written permission from your parents. If necessary, have the appropriate legal status so that there is no issue of your violating the confidentiality of a professional's relationship with your parent.

   Write down the questions you have before the meeting, and ask them. If the professionals do not take the time to answer your questions or if they do not make an appointment to spend the time you need, this may signal a problem. If the professionals are "too busy" to talk with you, you may wish to reexamine their appropriateness to your needs.

2. *Ask doctors and other specialists about books and other materials available to help you learn about particular problems or issues.*

3. *Even if you have a good primary care physician and appropriate medical specialists, remember that there are usually other individuals with expertise who can help you.* These include nonphysicians such as pharmacists, optometrists, and audiologists, as well as community specialists in family services, area agencies on aging, and home care services.

4. *Encourage your parents to have a positive attitude about themselves.* They are not just patients. They should be actively involved in their own medical care, family decisions, lifestyle choices, and housing. You and others may help, but they are partners in these ventures. Try to avoid taking over the decision making unless absolutely necessary.

5. *If necessary, be assertive!* Ask the professionals intelligent questions, and recognize whether you are getting accurate

responses or being brushed off. You will not be able to control things if you do not get the information you need. You can be assertive without being hostile or angry.

6. *Create an atmosphere of trust, respect, and communication.* Listen to what the professionals are saying to you. Do not be afraid of asking them to repeat or explain more clearly what you do not understand. Let people finish their thoughts before you interrupt them.

7. *Be polite and patient but persistent.* It is likely that you will need to speak with many professonals to get the information or help you need. Do not give up. Getting the right help requires doing good detective work.

A Special Note About Doctors

You may know that your parents have a good doctor just because you feel comfortable with them. But it is also not uncommon for adult children to be ill at ease, upset, or even irritated with their parents' physician. You may hear them saying "nothing can be done," "it is only old age," or something of that sort. Do not be afraid to ask for a second opinion, and find the second doctor from another source. If you have had bad experiences with a physician, or if you feel inhibited, shy, or otherwise unable to take advantage of their expertise, find someone you trust and who trusts you.

Knowing that you have a good physician to whom you can entrust the care of your parents is essential for your peace of mind. William Haley, Jeffrey Clair, and Karen Saulsberry, in their work in psychology and medical sociology of caregiving, have developed a survey to help caregivers judge the physicians caring for their aging parents. Read the following statements and think about whether any of them describe your experiences with your parents' doctor. Your answers may reveal how satisfied you are with them.

- The doctor gathered a detailed history from your parents and interviewed you as well.

- The doctor told you everything you and your parents wanted to know.

- The doctor seemed knowledgeable about your parents' problems.

- The doctor asked about all of your parents' current medications and their doses—why they were taking them, and what other professionals were involved in providing care.

- The doctor explained the purpose and results of medical tests.

- The doctor gave you a diagnosis or some explanation of your parents' problems.

- After talking with the doctor, you and your parents had a good idea of how serious the illness was—or was not.

- The doctor told you about all the available treatments.

- The doctor explained the illness in a way that you and your parents knew what to expect.

- The doctor thoroughly explained the purpose of the prescribed medications and how to take them.

- The doctor answered all your concerns.

- The doctor spent enough time with you and your parents.

- You felt understood by the doctor.

- The doctor made you feel that you were important—or at least did not brush you off as if you were merely a meddlesome intruder.

- The doctor gave you and your parents an opportunity to say what was on your minds.

- The doctor provided or suggested specific reading material about the medical problem.

- The doctor asked you how you were coping with the stress of caregiving.

- The doctor asked you and your parents for your thoughts on carrying out the medical treatments.

- The doctor acknowledged your contributions.

- You felt free to talk about family problems.

- The doctor made you feel like a competent caregiver.

- The doctor said he or she was not sure or knowledgeable about something and would check.

These questions are not intended to be scored. They are listed here to give you an opportunity to think about the experiences you have had with your parents' doctors. Your answers may help you decide that your parents need someone else, someone who cares about them and you.

ABOUT FINANCIAL PLANNING

Many health conditions can affect a person's ability to handle money matters. The increasing complexity of making financial decisions is one reason that financial and personal services are growing across the country to help older people pay their bills, read their mail, do their taxes, keep track of their insurance, and do routine bookkeeping as well as investment planning.

If you live close to your parents geographically, you may be able to help them. But if you live far away or if you do not want to get involved with their finances, call the agencies or organizations in Appendix C for assistance.

The following checklist can help you organize yourself to work with your parents on their financial situation. Keep this worksheet, and check it yearly to monitor their financial progress.

Many older people, particularly those with memory problems, are unduly influenced by people who find them easy prey and influence them financially, with tragic consequences. Fraud is often perpetrated on older persons. Knowing your parents' assets is the key to monitoring any untoward change in those assets. In some instances, contacting the State Attorney General may be necessary.

Assets (What They Own)

1. Retirement plan   _____
2. Total bank funds   _____
3. Other income investments (bonds, CDs, etc.)   _____
4. Common stocks, including mutual funds   _____
5. Real estate investment equity (market value)   _____
6. Other investments (business interest, collectibles, etc.)   _____
7. Net value of business   _____
8. Market value of home   _____
9. Cash value of life insurance   _____
10. Personal property, furniture, jewelry   _____
11. Automobile(s)   _____
12. Miscellaneous other assets (security deposits, money owed you)   _____
13. Total assets: 1–12   _____

Your Parents' Liabilities (What They Owe)

14. Balance on mortgage(s)   _____
15. Taxes due   _____
16. Automobile loans   _____
17. Other loans (e.g., home equity)   _____
18. Debt (e.g., credit cards)   _____
19. Total liabilities: Add lines 14–18   _____
20. Net worth: Subtract line 19 from line 13   _____

It may also help you to work with your parents to fill out a personal expense form. The following is a guide for your use.

Expenses	Current Year
1. Housing (mortgage, rent, taxes)	_____
2. Utilities (electricity, water, gas, oil, telephones, etc.)	_____
3. Transportation	_____
4. Repairs	_____
5. Food	_____
6. Payments	_____
7. Clothing	_____
8. Insurance (property, automobile, health, life)	_____
9. Repayments of credit cards, loans	_____
10. Recreation (entertainment, sports, hobbies)	_____
11. Vacation	_____
12. Miscellaneous expenses	_____
13. Savings and retirement investments	_____
14. Taxes (local, state, and federal)	_____
15. Contributions	_____
16. Total expenses: Add lines 1–15	_____

How to Deal with Conflicts in Partnerships

Have you ever been in any of the following situations?

- Your parents accuse you of not doing enough, even though you have visited them several times a week and done the best you can. *How can you keep calm and get through to your parents?*

- While talking with your boss about needing to take time off to help your father, she accuses you of not being productive enough to take off any more time. *How can you keep cool, care for your father, and still keep your job?*

- While you, your parents, and other members of your family are talking to the doctor, your brother interrupts you and criticizes you for a thought you have not been able to finish. *How can you respond without acting angry?*

- You are talking with your parents about the possibility of their moving into a retirement community. After you finish, both of them smile and politely say no. *What response from you will allow you to keep discussing the subject without turning them off?*

- You are talking with your parents' physician, who indicates that your father is just a nervous person and that there is no indication of an emotional problem. The lack of sleep, the weight loss, and the anxiety that your father manifests are only the result of his worry about a possible heart problem. You have good reason to think your father has a serious depression. *How do you confront the doctor without alienating him?*

These are only a few of the many possible confrontations, and you know how they make you feel. Most decisions in parent-caring involve negotiations. The questions for you to answer are: How effectively are you doing this? Can you learn to be more effective?

Whether you like it or not, you and your parents will need to negotiate with each other as well as with others for many different services, and you are likely to come into conflict with the people who help you. How well you handle such conflicts will affect not only whether you solve the problems but how good you feel about the solutions.

Negotiation is the art of getting what you want from people in a way that makes the best sense to both or all of you. In caregiving, you and your parents will want to share various things with each other—information, time, recognition, understanding, assistance with specific tasks, control, love, security, comfort, and a sense of accomplishment. You may also want many of these same things from health care, legal, and other professionals.

As we have already mentioned many times now, giving care while being caught up in multiple demands creates conflicts within you and between you and others. The way you approach resolving a conflict will have a significant impact on its outcome. Successful conflict resolution rests upon how well you recognize the potential harm of the conflict before it explodes, how confident you are in your abilities to deal with conflict situations, how well you understand your own style of dealing with interpersonal conflict, your level of insight into the expectations and interpersonal styles of the people with whom you are working, and your own conflict management and negotiation skills.

Examine Your Need to Negotiate

Read through the list below, and underline the words indicating individuals with whom you experience conflict. Then circle the degree of severity of conflict.

	Low	Medium	High
Mother	1	2	3
Father	1	2	3
Mother-in-law	1	2	3
Father-in-law	1	2	3
Brother(s)	1	2	3
Sister(s)	1	2	3
Children	1	2	3
Other relative(s)	1	2	3
Doctor(s)	1	2	3
Nurse(s)	1	2	3

Other health professional(s)	1	2	3
Chore worker	1	2	3
Home health aide	1	2	3
Homemaker	1	2	3
Co-workers	1	2	3
Other individuals			
_____	1	2	3
_____	1	2	3
_____	1	2	3
_____	1	2	3

If you have checked off two or more individuals with whom your conflict level is a 3, it will benefit you to examine the issues at stake as well as your negotiation skills. You can become a more successful negotiator if you are willing to try.

Tips for Successful Negotiations

Numerous books have been written by experts in negotiation and conflict resolution that can help you develop these skills. If you want to spend some time and energy to get really good, these books are worth studying. We have listed a few in the Selected Readings section at the back of this book. Reading will help you begin to deal constructively with those individuals or situations where conflict occurs.

1. *Accept that conflict is likely to occur whenever people are dealing with complex changes in their personal or business life.*
There are constructive ways to deal with conflict if you understand your objectives and if you can accept a successful resolution for all parties. Remember that conflict may develop as a natural response when people do not know how they fit into the greater picture. There is a story about three men who were laying bricks. When the first man was asked, "What are you doing?" he answered, "I'm laying bricks." The second man responded, "I'm building

a wall," and the third man said, "We are building a house of worship for our community." All were correct, but the third man was the best motivated to do well because he was the only one who kept in mind the ultimate purpose of what they were doing.

2. *The golden rule applies, albeit with a variation, to caregiving.* You need to understand the needs, wishes, and expectations of others. It seems clear, therefore, that you need to ask yourself the following questions: Why are the others involved? What are their needs and goals? Are these goals synchronous with mine? With each other? How do we differ? How much can we converge? How can I get people to realize that they need each other?

3. *Keep calm.* Do what you should do when you are in any stressful situation—take three deep breaths to regain control of yourself before you do anything! If you feel that you are getting into trouble, take "time out" to think about what to do before you rush to do it. A great deal of conflict occurs because people fly off the handle without thinking.

4. *Act as if you were coated in Teflon.* Be prepared to deal with the pain, but try not to let anything stick to you. When people are upset, they often say many disconcerting and often unintentional things. Do not dwell on them. Attribute them to the heat of the argument.

   Parents will criticize their children, and children will criticize their parents out of anguish. Let it pass, particularly if a parent has any brain disease, where abusive and foul language often occur. It is common for adult children in these situations to say, "I could not believe what I was hearing. I never thought that my mother even knew those words—how could she call me a ———? I don't think I'll ever get over it." Many people with brain damage such as from Alzheimer's disease cannot control their own reactions to frustration, stress, and rage. Their impulses overwhelm their self-control, and their emotions are no longer under their control. Their words come out in an exaggerated emotional way, often creating a vivid impression. Yet a few minutes later, it may seem as if nothing had been said. If you yourself lose control, take those deep breaths, back away, and then return and apologize. If your parents or others insult you, accept it and be prepared to "cool off" and refocus on solving the problem.

5. *Agree to disagree.* Not every problem has a solution that everyone will accept. If this is the case, try to redefine the problem to see if there is another way to help. If not, then agree to disagree.

6. *Accept that you may be vulnerable.* Without your realizing it, you may be the one who is engendering the conflict. Sometimes anger that is carried into a tense situation expresses itself through irritability, obstinacy, or angry words. Your hostility may be passive if you inadvertently throw a monkeywrench into a situation. Often the best way to deal with your own irritation is through humility.

   Interestingly enough, humility is not a bad approach to many problems. When you pray, for example, you are admitting your vulnerability and accepting that you are part of a larger universe. Remember that no matter what you do, you are part of a larger picture of meaning in life. Sometimes adopting this attitude can help you reduce your anger and deflect a potentially destructive and combative situation.

   One technique that can be effective is to find your place in nature. When you are caught up in very tense and difficult situations, try to go to a nearby window and gaze at some beauty of nature—realize that in another million years, the problem will be long forgotten, but the beauty of what you see will still prevail. Mountains, lakes, oceans, and plains all carry with them the important message that we and our problems fade into insignificance in the tapestry of our world. Putting your problems in this broader perspective can help.

Three Types of Action in Partnerships

If the overall goal is to take action in relation to others, different types of action are likely to be appropriate in different situations with different people. There are at least three basic styles of action when you are working with other people to care for your parents. One type of action is investigative: collecting information and finding services and programs to help. An emergency or crisis-oriented response is a second style of action when a serious problem occurs suddenly—an illness, an accident, or an urgent problem threatening someone's safety and well-being. A third type of action involves dealing with events and circumstances over the long term in practical ways.

Investigating a Problem

Finding information, however simple it may seem, is one of the most time-consuming tasks of caregivers. How do you find a good doctor, hospital, nursing home, retirement community, or community-based service? What services are available to help your parents live independently at home? How can you find out what Medicare and insurance policies cover? Where do you go for a good workup for your mother's many physical problems? How do you get information on multiple sclerosis, lupus, Alzheimer's disease, or any other disease, for that matter?

When you first recognize the existence of a problem, you need to get reliable information. If a doctor has given you a diagnosis, you may want a second opinion from a specialist. If your doctor has given your parent a diagnosis of Alzheimer's disease, you will need information about what might happen and how to organize your life around someone who will slowly but progressively deteriorate. Or if the doctor has told you that your parent has a very short time to live, you may wish to find out about hospice care or other alternatives. If your parents want to move into a retirement community, you will need to investigate the desirability and cost of various retirement homes.

Investigative activities are an important part of caregiving. Usually there is no easy way to get the necessary information, and

persistence and patience are probably the most important characteristics you will need. By planning and thinking through the issue, you will eventually find out what you need to know. If you give
up, the problem will only continue and you will become increasingly upset. The information you collect can be the basis for other
actions.

To locate the information you need, consider the following:

1. If your parent has a specific disease, locate a national
   organization that specializes in that disease, such as the
   Alzheimer's Disease Association, the American Cancer
   Society, or the American Heart Association. Call and
   ask about knowledgeable professionals and services in
   your area. The national offices of many of these organizations are listed in Appendixes C and D. Most of them
   have state or local offices, which can be helpful.

2. Every state has an agency on aging or elder affairs. Call
   your state offices (see Appendix B) and ask for a local
   number for this agency.

3. Ask your doctor or nurse for help or for advice on where to
   obtain information. You could also check with your local
   library.

4. See the Selected Readings section at the end of this book
   for pertinent material.

5. Plan ahead. Get the names and phone numbers of people and agencies in your community that are knowledgeable about caring for older persons. Keep them in
   a desk drawer. Having this practical information available in advance can save you time and aggravation in
   the future.

Emergency Action

Everyone has to face crises, whether they are accidents, illnesses,
or other emergencies at home, at work, or at school. In an emergency, events happen quickly and human lives may be at risk. The

situation usually appears unstable and unpredictable. Some form of action is needed quickly to contain or remove the danger.

The following are characteristics of emergencies:

- There is a threat of danger or harm.
- The situation is unstable and unpredictable.
- The situation progresses rapidly.
- Urgent action is required.
- The situation is very emotional.

The guidelines below can help you in emergency situations.

1. Evaluate the situation as accurately as you can. Get others to confirm your assessment, if possible. Do not rely on rumor.

2. Try to determine what might happen if things remain unchecked.

3. Assess the potential dangers to the people directly involved.

4. Focus your attention. Determine who and what needs to be involved to assist and to make decisions, and do not spend much time with people or issues that are not directly related to the emergency.

5. Avoid taking actions for their own sake. Some of them may make things worse. Do not act on emotional impulses without information that supports your action.

6. Decide on a strategy, but be prepared to change it if it is not working.

7. Reevaluate the situation periodically, even if nothing new seems to have happened.

8. Do not panic, and do not let others panic.

9. If you cannot control your feelings and actions, find someone who can do what needs to be done.

Practical Action

The principle in practical action is to use your common sense and figure out what you can reasonably do. Pragmatic action can involve small, helpful behaviors: You see what needs to be done, and you do it! Your mother is lying in the hospital bed with dried food on her lips, so you take a wet cloth and wipe it off. Your father is moving slowly toward the elevator with his walker, so you ask someone to hold the door open till he gets in. These minor, seemingly obvious behaviors all come together as a style of action to make things happen. Being pragmatic means being sensitive to situations and to the people involved in them to do what seems right.

Being pragmatic leads to being effective—getting things done. It means using what resources you have to do what needs doing, or if you do not have the resources, doing everything you can with what you have while arranging to get what is needed. Throughout the course of parent-caring, it is a good habit to ask yourself periodically, What is my most effective course of action?

Doing the *right* thing, at minimum, means taking the initiative and the responsibility to get involved. If your first response does not work, you need to be flexible and find another. There is not always a single, fixed way to do a task, and sometimes doing nothing but wait is the appropriate action. You need to keep your cool and make practical decisions as you go along. Indeed, this may be the time to put down all the books you have read and follow your intuition, based on your sensitivities.

The following is a list of steps for pragmatic action:

1. Assess the situation: What is wrong, what needs to happen, and who can help?

2. Do whatever is reasonable to make things better, and get help if possible.

3. Take the initiative. Do not wait for a perfect answer.

4. Keep your self-control.

5. Watch for changes in the situation.

6. Be flexible. Change your tactics if you need to do so.

7. Keep the long haul in mind. One of the secrets to successful long-distance running is to pace yourself. Solve the immediate problem, but remember the longer-term goals. Think about the need to reserve your resources as you act to solve problems today.

THE LONG HAUL

Creating and maintaining partnerships means caring for yourself and others over the long haul. The fine art of caring requires that you discover ways to increase your effectivity—your ability to meet everyone's needs as you work through the many challenges of caregiving. You will be buffeted by many forces as you try to keep yourself on track. The next chapter describes how you can learn the skills of effectivity for balancing the needs of your parents and others in your family.

5

BALANCING NEEDS
AND RESOURCES

There is no crash course that can teach you how to be an effective caregiver. And a crash course would be exactly the wrong strategy in any case. Effectivity is a long-term pursuit, as you learn what works for you through the acquisition of information and the experience of doing. There is a body of knowledge about strategies for taking effective action, and time is on your side to learn it because parent-caring often goes on for many years. You will experience periods of success when you are able to balance the needs of your parents, yourself, and others in your family. It is likely you also will experience periods when you are less successful in juggling everything that needs to be done.

Caring for parents often feels like an endless series of insurmountable problems because the number and magnitude of the problems feel so overwhelming, and you may not see that help is available. Your parents may have difficult personalities. Your own life may be demanding with work, family, and personal obligations. The story of Melissa Adams illustrates the incredible pressures and intricacies of trying to meet the needs of everyone in a family, as well as the challenge of maintaining effectivity in caregiving when the pressures last a long time and involve many people.

We start with a letter that Melissa wrote to her mother after she was unable to attend her mother's funeral. It is part of a daily diary she kept, with entries addressed to her mother.

Dear Mom,

It's 1:00 P.M., and my heart is breaking because I can't be with you. The doctors won't let me leave the hospital, and my body is in pretty sad shape after the spinal surgery.

So I'm writing this to say good-bye. I asked our minister to read my favorite poem from your last book at the grave so you would know I was with you.

It must feel good to be free from that awful Alzheimer's disease that tore you apart over the years. I hope you find peace now that it's over.

Check heaven out, because Bobbie should be joining you soon. You never knew he had AIDS, which is the only good thing the Alzheimer's disease did for you. It saved you from watching your youngest son die.

Mom, I miss you so much now. I'm glad your anguish is over, but it hurts to know I'll never see you again. You always gave me so much strength, and I need you more than ever now.

Melissa wrote this in an effort to deal with powerful emotions that were overwhelming her. For years afterward, she continued to keep the diary, describing it as her "survival manual." She needed it to maintain her sanity through the years of sickness and death in her family—her brother Bobbie's AIDS, her mother's Alzheimer's disease, her sister's cancer, her father's stroke, her husband's drinking problem, and her own struggle to recover from two operations on her spine.

Melissa had been an extremely effective caregiver. After her mother, Charlotte Sarton, developed Alzheimer's disease, Melissa inherited Mrs. Sarton's role as the emotional center of the family. She was very much like her mother—and she became the one who looked after everyone. Even when Melissa went into the hospital for spinal surgery, she had everything organized. She arranged for someone to take care of her father, her brother Bobbie, and her sister Marcie. Melissa attributed her capacity to care for everyone to her mother's influence:

Mom was my strength, and even though she is dead, she is still my model. Her spirit is very much alive! I write to her every day—and I often talk out loud to her. . . . I know she is listening. I need her there to sort things out. . . . Mom is the only one to listen to me now. Everyone else is sick!

Most of her immediate family were very sick. Her father continued to live at home after his stroke, with a homemaker and weekly home nursing visits. Marcie had been given a forty-sixty chance of surviving her brain tumor. And Bobbie's AIDS was breaking her heart.

Following her own surgeries, Melissa needed help with almost everything—bathing, dressing, going to the bathroom, and just getting around. She had many good friends who pitched in to help her recover. Melissa was easy to care for except one thing—her unending conversations with her mother. Melissa's "talks" with her mother were frightening to her friends because she seemed to be retreating into a world of make-believe.

Melissa knew that her obsession with her mother's memory was not helpful to her anymore. It had become a way to escape from her pain and dilute her grief over the many tragedies in her family. Holding on to her mother had been an emotional anchor for Melissa, who had always been able to handle everything and everyone. Now, for the first time, she was tired, sick, and unable to move forward. Looking after everyone during the seven years since her mother first got sick had sapped her strength. Melissa was convinced that she had become vulnerable to the spinal meningitis precisely because she was so run down. She had read that stress affects the immune system, and she wondered if she would have gotten sick at all if she had taken better care of herself.

Melissa had taken care of herself in the beginning, and she had worked closely with her mother. Indeed, Melissa had appeared to be doing all the right things. She had felt strongly that it was important for her mother to "call the shots" from the beginning. During the many hours that Melissa spent with her mother, sitting in offices waiting for diagnostic tests, the two of them talked about the future and what they would do if Mrs. Sarton had something like Alzheimer's disease.

The morning the doctor confirmed their worst fears, Melissa

took her mother out to lunch. Melissa knew how scared her mother was. The memory losses had been affecting the role she valued so highly. Mrs. Sarton had always taken care of everyone else, and she knew that someday she would not be able to do this. Melissa described their lunch conversation this way:

> I told Mom that she was still the center of the family, and I would help her stay in the center. She had helped me in so many ways that it was only fair that she let me give something back.
>
> We agreed to call a family meeting over dinner to talk about her future. It was important to Mom that she do the entire meal, although she wanted me there to keep her company. . . . She called it her last supper.
>
> I trembled when I heard "my last supper." She laughed at me and said she needed to deal with this disease her way. This would be her meal—not one prepared by someone else. Before she got much worse, she wanted to do one of the things that brought her great pleasure—cooking for everyone.

That family dinner marked the beginning of what Mrs. Sarton called "living with the A word." The family was too upset about her diagnosis that first night to even begin to talk about a coherent plan. It would take several meetings together, as well as a long visit with the doctor, to understand what it meant to live with Alzheimer's disease.

From the very beginning, Melissa assumed the executive and managerial roles. She was the one who brought the family together, shared the information from the doctors, helped identify the problems, and prodded others to come up with suggestions. Trying to get the rest of the family involved was not without difficulty. Melissa was the oldest of four children. Although she had good relationships with Marcie and her other brother, Arnold, both expressed mild resentment that Melissa seemed to be "taking over." This issue surfaced early in the family meeting, first as questioning some of the decisions, then questioning even the diagnosis. "Don't we need another opinion?" asked Marcie, who proposed that yet another workup be done "just in case they missed something." Questions about the course of the illness and what should be done came out in a challenging way. Finally, when Mrs. Sarton left the room, Marcie blurted out, "Tell me how come you're in charge all of a sudden," to her sister. Arnold, trying not to take sides between his two sisters, nonetheless seemed to be wondering the same thing.

Melissa felt hurt, but she was careful not to defend herself or attack Marcie, although this was her first impulse. She wanted to involve her siblings in the care of her mother and reduce rather than enhance her responsibilities. She explained to Marcie:

> Mom and I called this meeting precisely to deal with this issue. We have spent more time together over the years for a lot of reasons, so Mom asked me to take her to the doctors and I got to talk with them. I didn't consciously "cut" you and Arnold out, and that is the furthest thing from my mind—that's why I called you every time I learned something. But I guess I may sound controlling because I am telling you what they said.

When she returned, Mrs. Sarton took over:

> There is so much I want to do before my mind goes away completely. All of you mean so much to me, and I need you around me to beat this disease. Maybe Melissa has become close, but that is because we have spent so much time together.
>
> But that doesn't mean I love Melissa more than you. I know Melissa better than you. Before my mind goes away, I want us all to become a closer family again. There is so little time left!

Even the most loving, loyal, and cooperative families experience tensions somewhere along the way. Melissa knew that her sister's feelings were based on a long-standing jealousy, but she also knew that those feelings should not interfere with the greater problem—their mother's needs. One of the hardest tasks for Melissa and the others was to set limits on what each could and should do. Melissa described her feelings this way:

From the very beginning I felt guilty that I couldn't do enough for Mom. It was our minister who finally helped me see that I shouldn't feel guilty. I was doing the best I could. I was meeting most of her needs.

My problem was me. . . . I expected myself to do more. The guilt feelings came because I thought I should be able to do everything, and that just wasn't possible.

A special meeting took place with their minister, Reverend Carter, but without Mrs. Sarton so that Melissa and the family could talk honestly about their feelings and responsibilities to their mother. Ever since the diagnosis everyone had felt that they had to be with her as much as possible. Although the family had always done things together, somehow this was different. Reverend Carter observed that the family was acting as if Mrs. Sarton were dying or already incompetent and could not be alone. They had put their lives on hold to be with her all the time. Reverend Carter suggested that from what he knew about Alzheimer's disease, it could be years before Mrs. Sarton was so debilitated that she would need constant help.

The minister also opened the door to frank discussions about the fact that Mrs. Sarton was likely to get worse—something none of them wanted to think or talk about. Everyone was deeply grieved and could not deal with their fear and anxieties. Melissa described it this way:

I felt as if we could keep her from getting worse if we stayed close and protected her. I really couldn't accept that she had Alzheimer's disease. I thought she just needed more stimulation . . . and to keep active.

Now I can see that we were acting in a crazy way. We actually were making things worse. If it hadn't been for Reverend Carter, we might have ended up so burned out, angry, and frustrated that when Mom really needed us, we might not have been able to help!

Our family learned an important lesson—to measure out the care as Mom needs it, not as we need to show our love for her or meet our own needs. We were doing everything for her because we hurt so much, and we lost our perspective.

For several years Melissa worked closely with her mother and the rest of the family as Mrs. Sarton slowly deteriorated. Then the sequence of family tragedies left Melissa to bear the burden alone. She managed to carry on for a while, but eventually the demands of caring coupled with her own poor health were incapacitating.

Melissa's situation illustrates the single greatest risk of caregiving: If you do it long enough and intensively enough without managing your effectivity, you have a high probability of endangering your own health. Over time, the demands of coping with chronic problems and the pileup of life stresses can lead to serious physical and mental health problems, unless you develop realistic strategies to protect yourself. In the next chapter we describe how you can recognize when you are in danger of losing control. The purpose of this chapter is to discuss guidelines to help you develop and maintain your effectivity.

FOUR GUIDELINES TO IMPROVE YOUR CARING BEHAVIOR

1. Take a close look at your family—needs and problems— but mainly its strengths.

2. Find ways to establish good communication with family members, and spend the time doing it.

3. Assess the situation from the perspective of everyone involved—get everyone's input at family meetings.

4. Identify tasks and formulate plans.

These constitute a general approach to increase effective caring, but they will need to be modified and implemented depending on your own situation. Every family and every situation are different, and what works for you may not work for someone else. Not all families will be able to have successful meetings to deal with caregiving responsibilities. Not everyone has a family to rely upon, and it is not always possible to get your parents involved in decision making. You will need to judge how much you can or should expect from other family members. And if your expectations are not met, it is important to understand why. The pressures of caring may lead you to press others for involvement, but they may resist because they are scared or because they do not feel it is their responsibility.

Expect to be criticized by your family members for whatever you do! It is quite common. You may believe that you have done something helpful, only to have your jealous brothers and sisters describe you as a villain. Their allegations may range from mistreatment to abuse to financial skulduggery. These are some of the hardest times to prevent yourself from losing control. Recognize that such accusations are the emotional outbursts of upset relatives expressing their frustration and impotence at not being able to change the reality of a problem. Find a way to retain your composure, and offer to share the burden with them or ask them to suggest a better plan of care.

If your family members stay away, resist involvement, or criticize you at every turn, it may be a pattern of reacting that they developed during previous family crises. The way people behave toward one another develops over time. If brothers and sisters have been distant and uninvolved in family life or jealous about parental favoritism in the past, it should not be surprising that when aged parents require assistance, they are unwilling or difficult partners. If other family members are hostile and adamantly opposed to your suggestions, think twice before creating a scene. Inducing guilt or pressing for help is more likely to cause anger and complicate your life further. You may be better off "cutting your losses" and finding help outside the family.

YOUR FAMILY AFFECTS YOUR EFFECTIVENESS

Before you take any actions to develop a plan, you need to have a sense of how your family operates, as we have emphasized throughout this book. A plan developed in one family may not work in another because people are so different. Not every family works well together or even wants to work together. Moreover, to be effective you need to understand the talents, liabilities, and availability of everyone who is or might be involved. The size and composition of your family; factors like divorce, geographical distance, economics, and previous conflicts; as well as the willingness and ability of family members to help each other all influence your effectiveness in family problem solving. The important issue here is for you to develop reasonable expectations of your family based upon the way the family works. Everyone should be given an opportunity to participate, but how they participate can be negotiated. It may be more effective not to involve any family members who do not want to help or who obstruct your efforts, but this should not be a personal decision for you to make—share it with others.

Family Styles

There are five general ways or styles in which most families solve problems: denial, cooperation, alternating leadership, contentiousness, and chaos. Families characterized by strong *denial* do not see a problem coming in advance and act as if nothing were going wrong when it arrives. People are hard to mobilize in such families, and planning is a problem. Yet these families seem to be constantly in a state of crisis, since the situations they do face are those that have gotten so serious that denial is no longer possible and rapid emergency action is required.

Families with a *cooperative* style seek to confront and solve collaboratively the challenges that beset them. They are usually effective working together and sharing their burdens. This is in part because they maintain open communication and cooperation.

The third family style is one where members *alternate leadership* rather than collaborate with one another. Things go well as long as the family members agree about who will take charge during specified periods. Arguments over leadership can be toxic and can split such families with acrimony.

The fourth family style is *contentiousness*, or a long history of family feuds and disagreements. It seems impossible for members of such families to work together on anything. Some have described this family style as crabs in a barrel; when one person moves up, the others pull it down. Anger is pervasive, and insecurity and conflict abound. Professionals try to shy away from such families because they perceive so much "nastiness."

Finally, some families are simply *chaotic*. Relationships in such families are so disorganized and so embittered that parent-caring becomes one more vehicle by which members hurt each other. In some chaotic families, members have little hostility for one another but simply are not connected, like a pile of spare parts rather than an effective machine.

These five styles may sound as if every family can be typed in black-and-white terms. Obviously, this is not the case! Few families are so cooperative that there is no discord, or so chaotic that older relatives get ignored or abused. Families often show combinations of these styles. Some families may appear to be contentious and bitter, but when something life-threatening happens, a consensus emerges as a basis for cooperative decisions about the best way to proceed. Other families may start out being superficially cooperative—until problems ensue that necessitate real sacrifices. At that point serious family rifts emerge, destroying the decision-making process. Wills and inheritances are issues that have the potential to create family warfare, where greed becomes a sad but real problem with families.

You do not have to have a degree in psychology to understand your family's style. You should, however, try to recall past events—hopefully without too much emotion—and use this perspective to get some leverage on the present. If serious denial, belligerence, contentiousness, and angry chaotic behaviors have been present in your family, you may wish to think about getting help for your family early on. This does not necessarily mean professional help, but you will need others, such as friends or clergy, to act as referees. If you reach the conclusion that your family cannot work together at all, it will be in your best interest to avoid the headaches of trying to involve them, except as necessary. You may be better off doing things without them after initially trying to involve them—keep them informed without expecting any thanks for what you do. Indeed, their anger may be your only reward beyond your internal satisfaction that you have done the right thing.

If you run into very serious problems and your relatives are making your life difficult, get professional help! Unfortunately, it is all too common for a caregiving family member to be accused of trying to take over a parent's estate or assets—by the same siblings who stood on the sidelines for years, doing nothing to help. This may be a traumatic experience, especially when your own brother or sister is the antagonist. You may need to find a helpful attorney specializing in family law.

The sad reality is that such behavior does occur. One of the important reasons for families to come together early in the process of parent-caring is to focus on the question of finances. This discussion should address concerns about the estate of your parents. Banks are now offering "reverse mortgages," in which the value of a property is credited toward a monthly income, in exchange for the home after the death of the owner. (See the Selected Readings section at the back of the book for more information on this and other options.)

Whatever your family situation, you will need to practice communicating with one another. The following guidelines may help you.

How to Establish Effective Family Communication

Frequently we do not say what we mean, or we do not hear exactly what someone else means. As discussed at length in Chapter 3, our emotions cloud our ability to listen and think clearly, and we often react based upon our feelings rather than our thoughts. Not surprisingly, conflicts often erupt over unnecessary misunderstandings. Tensions may revive longstanding power struggles among family members, and when this happens, communication deteriorates.

Learning to be an effective communicator requires preparation and practice. Decide what you want to say—and then simplify it. You can add supplementary information later as needed to prove your points and answer questions. You can also write out the points you want to make before the meeting.

It is also very helpful to practice "active listening." Active listening means making an effort to understand the underlying message or meaning of what another person is saying, and then checking to see if you have correctly interpreted what was said. This technique is useful to avoid jumping to conclusions about what someone is saying because you are too busy rehearsing your own response to receive an accurate message in the first place.

Active listening means concentrating on the speaker's words as well as on the feelings behind the words. One way to do this is to close your eyes and listen to the tone of the speaker's voice—its volume and inflections. Or watch a person's body language, and see if the words and voice match the way they hold themselves and behave.

Active listening does not always work, but it is a valuable tool. There are several ways you can set the stage for active listening and effective communication during family discussions.

1. Ask people to speak one at a time without interrupting each other. We frequently interrupt each other when we are anxious, upset, or angry. Encourage people to make their points as clearly as possible, then ask them to listen closely to what the others say. If someone must say something, they should ask permission. Furthermore, when someone is long-winded, interrupt them politely and ask them to summarize their main points, indicating that they will have more time to speak after others have presented their arguments.

2. Encourage people to speak for themselves and not for others. We often make assumptions about what other people think, feel, and want. It is important not to do this, especially for someone who is sick. All too often spouses and children try to speak for an older relative. Although family members can be helpful interpreters and advocates, they can also undermine the process of finding out what the older person really needs and wants.

Family members often unknowingly act as if their parents want the same thing they do. It is normal to act this way, but it can make things worse rather than better. It is not fair to simply endow others with one's own beliefs. Your family should make decisions with respect to the parents' comfort, safety, well-being, and dignity from their own point of view rather than yours or any other individual's. While it is important for everyone to share ideas and reactions, it is also important to identify who is speaking for whom and about whom.

3. Ask people to distinguish as clearly as they can between facts and opinions and between thoughts and feelings. This is hard work because it means concentrating and thinking about what we are saying. At the time of her diagnosis Mrs. Sarton had only mild memory problems and a little difficulty finding the right words. But her husband, who was alive at the time, was terrified, although he was afraid to admit it, and he could only focus on how sick she was. He could not separate his own emotional reactions to her diagnosis from her actual condition, which at the time of her diagnosis was pretty good. It was Angela, Melissa's daughter, who helped her grandfather: "Grandpa, Gram is not sick yet. I want you to stop crying and take a good look at her. She's pretty, and we are all going to help her and love her!"

Sometimes problems arise because facts and opinions are confused. Is a professional opinion the same as a fact? Is legal advice an opinion? Is the cost of care projected forward for a year a fact or an assumption? Each of these must be considered independently. Is the medical opinion a guess, or is it based upon a careful evaluation and laboratory tests leading to a firm diagnosis? What other options did the attorney provide under the relevant laws? What are the assumptions underlying the cost projection?

Separating fact from opinion means getting beyond mere statements of belief to learn what those opinions and beliefs are resting upon. Behavior should be based on the best knowledge at the time the decision was made. If later a decision seems to go awry, you can take comfort in knowing that, given the information available at the time, the decision was appropriate and correct—and given the same situation today, the decision might be the same.

4. Encourage people to avoid generalities and talk about specifics. Working toward a solution means getting down to brass tacks. It is easy to get hung up on the enormity of the problem and feel that you do not know what to do. Problem solving often requires considerable mental effort to force oneself to focus and concentrate on the details. Melissa's sister Marcie and her husband were overwhelmed by the prospect of Alzheimer's disease. Marcie could talk only about how upset she was and remark that there was nothing anyone could do. It was Mrs. Sarton who finally broke this emotional impasse: "I know this is hard on you and everyone else—but I'm the one who has the A word. Unless you can face up to it, you won't be able to help me—and I need all the help I can get!"

5. When different opinions emerge, encourage people to clarify their differences rather than argue about them. When legitimate concerns surface, they should be considered and given credibility. Arguments are sometimes unavoidable, but they can be destructive if the emotions that come out of them dominate the scene and delay your problem solving. When unresolvable issues emerge, they should be recognized as such and dropped. It is usually more effective to "agree to disagree" about some things and then try to work around the impasse. Angry confrontations often take on a life of their own and act like a fuse on a stick of dynamite, igniting emotional outbursts and escalating the impact of the nonproductive, underlying issues.

6. Encourage everyone to participate in the discussion in some way. Some family members need to be encouraged to contribute what may be valuable information to a problem-solving discussion. When everyone participates, even for a few moments, it establishes a sense of shared involvement and shared responsibility for the future. Likewise, it avoids the problem of the nonparticipant who says nothing but at the end of the meeting disagrees with the conclusions and works to undermine the consensus. Before ending the meeting, go around the room asking everyone by name if they have anything to add. Do not wait too long to do this, otherwise people may leave or be too tired to participate well. If too many have "cut out," then defer decision making to another meeting.

7. If you are leading the family discussion, try to understand and deal with your own emotions. In order to prepare yourself to guide the family discussion, you need to evaluate the role your sick relative is currently playing in the family, compared to their prior role as a healthier individual. It may be helpful to make two lists. One list should contain your emotional reactions to your relative before they became frail or sick, and the other should contain your current reactions. This exercise may seem silly and difficult, but it can help you understand how hard it is to analyze your feelings. As a group leader you will need to listen to yourself as well as to everyone else in the family, and it is essential that you not let your own feelings contaminate your behavior while you have responsibility for leading the discussions.

8. *Invite a close family friend to observe the meeting.* An outsider can be a useful observer and analyst of family behavior, and when the meeting is over this person can help you understand what took place and how people behaved. There are risks as well as gains when an observer joins the family. Relatives who know the observer less well may feel threatened and avoid talking about painful or emotional issues. Instead of listening and observing, a visitor may talk and disrupt family discussions. Well-intentioned but insensitive friends may provoke unnecessary family conflict by taking sides, or they may prematurely halt a disagreement rather than let it play itself out to its conclusion. If you do involve others, choose them carefully and emphasize to them, in private as well as publicly, that they need to be impartial and to listen.

GETTING EVERYONE'S PERSPECTIVE AT FAMILY MEETINGS

Family meetings should be called as frequently as they are necessary when it is possible to solicit everyone's perspective. But it is important to organize each meeting. Review the guidelines for communication at the beginning of the meeting. Ask the group to agree that they will abide by them during the meeting. Structure is more easily proposed than adhered to so keeping the discussion on track is critical. Setting a time to begin and end the meeting may help expedite things.

Discussion Leader

Even if it is you who convenes the meeting, you must be prepared to let the group nominate someone else to lead the discussion if they choose. Do not allow yourself to see this as a rejection. Remember that the cardinal rule for being effective is to focus on the goals, not on yourself.

It is important that you accept another leader as comfortably as possible. Allowing yourself to feel rejected—as opposed to relieved or gratified—is harmful. As hard as it may be, try not to jump to rapid, unfounded conclusions that the family does not want your leadership. In this situation as in many others, it is important to "go with the flow" of the group. Sometimes you are better able to influence what happens by working as a peer in addressing the situation.

You are not being displaced from your leadership role if another discussion leader is elected. In fact, there are many benefits to having someone else run the meeting. You can observe and distinguish the different points of view more thoughtfully, and you can see how your parents are reacting to what is being said. You can express your position more clearly, without appearing to be using your position as leader to force a specific agenda. If your relatives perceive that you are doing this, their resentment of you will defeat even your good ideas.

Focus

Structuring the meetings will help keep family members focused on the tasks of caregiving. Although a good discussion requires focus, this does not mean that conflict, disagreements, and feelings should be discouraged. Giving people the opportunity to vent their anger and frustrations is healthy. When many family members are involved, it is likely that they will disagree. The general agreement should be that such disagreements will not be permitted to get out of control.

It is difficult to keep a group of relatives focused on anything, much less problem solving, but if everyone agrees in advance to work at it the outcome will be to accept the idea of shared goals

and responsibility and some type of assignment and pooling of resources.

Sibling Rivalries

Discussions are likely to be and are sidetracked when old rivalries,
loyalties, or conflicts emerge. Sibling rivalries persist far beyond
childhood, and it is common for older brothers and sisters to get
caught up in competitive issues whose roots are in the early school
years, and thereby delay the resolution of parents' problems today.

Every so often, adult children use the illness or frailty of a
parent as an opportunity to renegotiate a longstanding problem
with the parent or to win an old battle with other members of the
family. This can become a serious problem when the dependent
older person is viewed as an object to be "owned" or controlled.
The adult children may vie with one another or with the other
parent to solve the problem "their" way, and these situations can
get hostile. It is almost like a battle over a family heirloom, unrelated to monetary value—objects such as a set of silver or china or
a collection of any sort that had a special emotional value can
catalyze conflict.

If hostility erupts during a family meeting and a mediator
is not present, the group leader might call a "time out," asking
everyone to take a break to regain their composure. When the
meeting reconvenes, restate the issue that started the conflict,
summarize the opposing arguments, and figure out how to achieve
some compromise. Sometimes a "time out" break allows people to
cool off enough to deal with the real issues of parent-caring. If the
discussion leader is closely identified with one side of the conflict,
it is a good idea to get someone less polarized to deal with the
consensus. If family warfare erupts without a mediator, try to stop
the meeting by asserting that an impasse has been reached and an
arbitrator is needed. Try to prevent harsh language and confrontations that can open up old wounds or create new ones.

Anxiety

Sometimes the anger that is expressed is due to anxiety and fear of
the future. When a family member is in trouble and others want to

help but do not know what to do, anxiety and uneasiness are natural responses even in healthy families. Anxiety is not necessarily bad, and in modest quantities it can be an energizer pushing the group forward. When anxiety levels are high, they inhibit communication and prevent the family from developing an effective resolution of important issues. One way you can deal with group anxiety effectively is to state openly that you know people are anxious and concerned and ask them to talk about what is making them anxious. If everyone can share their feelings, they may well begin to feel a sense of relief.

Family meetings do not always work. Strong emotions and old family battles may be too strong and create an impasse to problem solving. The family style may make a meeting impossible since most members might be "too busy to attend" or unwilling to share in the prospective caring. For some families, if there is a meeting, disruption is predictable. For such families it is imperative to get outside help—from a psychiatrist, psychologist, or social worker—who has experience working with families. It is a sign of strength for a family to recognize that it needs outside resources to break a serious impasse. The objective here is not to resolve long-standing family conflicts but to focus on what can realistically be done to meet the needs of the ailing parents.

In general, the more you engage other family members in the process of planning, the greater your chances of coming up with viable solutions. Furthermore, you are likely to discover more resources than you imagined as others become involved in the process. The family will also begin to build a collective sense of responsibility by sharing their options and ideas. Your solutions may not be perfect, but since they evolved from the collective efforts of the group, they offer something to build on.

IDENTIFY THE TASKS AND FORMULATE YOUR PLANS

Deciding what you want to accomplish can be overwhelming precisely because caring responsibilities feel so overwhelming. But establishing specific goals is essential if you and your family are to work together. In this sense, family problem solving is a lot like working on a jigsaw puzzle. You need to keep a mental picture of the puzzle in mind to put the pieces together more rapidly.

In addition, or as an alternative to some of the techniques already described, an effective tactic is to turn the family meeting into a work session. Give the family members pencil and paper and ask them to disperse and find a comfortable place to work. Ask them to spend about a half-hour developing a plan to respond to the situation at hand. When they reassemble, read the plans aloud and agree on segments that need to be taken care of. Then get an individual or a small group to address them.

This exercise is not a panacea, but it does provide everyone with "alone" time to come up with their own solutions or perspectives. Private time is essential because each person needs to figure out where they think the family should go. When people reconvene, they will be able to provide some thoughtful perspective. Even if family members resist doing this, encourage them to try.

Becoming more effective involves identifying the tasks that lie ahead. You can expect at least four broad sets of tasks that are associated with parent-caring to emerge: providing direct assistance to your aging parents, working with family members on interpersonal tasks, dealing with health and social professionals and agencies, and meeting your own personal needs. It is helpful to go over with the family the specific tasks that are likely to need attention. The list below is not meant to be exhaustive but rather a way to anticipate and discuss plans for care.

Direct Assistance Tasks

Since chronically ill individuals require assistance over long periods of time, the tasks and services required will change over time.

- Ask your parents to let you or someone else in the family obtain needed information from their doctor or other health professional.

- Get accurate information about your parents' problem or condition; particularly address their ability to perform the functions of daily living.

- Develop a partnership with your parents and with their health professionals to evaluate the options for treatment strategies.

- Supervise the daily administration of medical and other treatments.

- Supervise general health recommendations regarding diet, exercise, and other lifestyle changes.

- Find community services.

- Where possible, work with your parents to structure their daily activities in a meaningful way.

- Help with bathing, dressing, eating, walking, and any other personal care activities.

- Find help to deal with upsetting behaviors such as agitation, behavioral outbursts, and so on.

- Find ways to maintain a satisfying relationship with your parents.

- Find a time and place for enjoyment.

- Develop a mechanism to assist with your parents' finances, when appropriate.

- Evaluate the continuing ability of your parents to participate in their care.

- Anticipate your parents' needs for future assistance and services.

For each item on this list there are specific tasks that need to be performed. If help with personal hygiene, food purchases, or food preparation is needed, then decisions need to be made as to whether a homemaker should be hired or a relative should be made responsible for such chores. What is the backup plan? Who will pay if services are purchased?

Finding community services involves contacting social agencies to find one or more that can help with problems like yours. Companionship is often a shared family responsibility, but having a dozen relatives visiting for the same two hours does not constitute twenty-four hour coverage, if that is needed.

Remember that many families have members or close friends who are trained professionals. Do not be shy about involving them with the clinicians who are providing services to your parents.

Interpersonal Tasks with Other Family Members

It is difficult to be specific about performing discrete tasks with other family members because family relationships vary so much depending upon who you are, where you live, and how people work together. But certain tasks transcend these issues.

- Maintain family communication, exchanging information as you get it.

- Find ways to share responsibilities.

- Deal with negative feelings toward family members who do not help very often or at all.

- Make plans to deal with angry conflicts or rifts in the family when they have a negative impact on caregiving.

- When possible, discuss as a family the need for institutionalization before it becomes necessary. What is necessary to prevent it? Under what circumstances would it be a good idea? How would you find an acceptable facility?

Community Tasks

Much of what older people need lies in the realm of social and community services rather than medical interventions.

- Learn about social and other human services in your community.

- Make contacts with others who are knowledgeable.

- Explore alternative housing arrangements.

- Become an advocate for your parents.

Personal Tasks

Last but hardly least, you need to identify our own needs and to take care of yourself. The following is only a partial list of the tasks you will face. Remember, if you do not care for yourself, you are very likely to develop problems, and those problems can incapacitate you, ultimately harming your parents as well. Therefore, sage advice is that you arrange care for yourself—not for selfish reasons, although you deserve it—but as a responsibility for those who depend upon you. Take care of yourself!

- Find personal time away from your parents. Schedule it! Do it every day, if possible, for a couple of hours.

- Get enough sleep.

- Eat properly.

- Exercise and keep fit.

- Separate any angry feelings toward your parents from your angry feelings associated with the pressures of caregiving.

- Feel good about what you are doing.

- Find healthy ways to release your tensions.

- Learn to live one day at a time.

- Prepare for the uncertainty of progressive deterioration and death, but do not let hope die too far ahead of your parents.

- Talk with others; make time for friends.

- Make time for tenderness and affection with those you love.

- Confide in someone.

Making a list of the four kinds of tasks should bring a sense of relief to the family that caregiving involves specific activities rather than an overwhelming and amorphous situation. The key element is something we have stressed throughout the book: Take control! Take a deep breath, and examine how you and others will need to redefine your roles and obligations around caregiving responsibilities. Theodore Roosevelt said, "Do what you can, with what you have, where you are." And that is exactly what you need to do for continuing effectivity.

Your effectiveness, and the quality of your life and everyone else's requires that you and your family continue to monitor the situation—evaluate changes in your parents and changes in the family—reevaluate the best course of action under changing circumstances, then do what needs to be done. Except in rare circumstances—when a parent's life is in imminent danger—you have the time to develop and carry out your plan. The next chapter describes how you can reduce your risk of losing control and how to recognize when you or others in your family may be heading for trouble.

6

TAKING CONTROL
IN A CRISIS

It is the rare family where plans are implemented smoothly and changes occur without some conflict or upset. Even if you have coped well with most of the demands of caregiving, there may be times when you feel that you are reaching your breaking point. A personal experience may cause you to need to blow off steam, or a family experience may make tensions run high and cause arguments to break out. In these situations you may lose control and say or do stupid, hurtful things. How many times have you said something in anger to someone that you later wished you could retract? Even loving brothers and sisters fight with each other.

No matter how devoted you are to your parents or spouse, you will have disagreements over something. Healthy people in healthy families experience conflicts and disruptions that are usually short-lived. Serious problems, however, may erupt in families when the demands of caregiving outstrip the family's abilities and resources, when family relationships have been disruptive or unpleasant for a long period of time, or when crises pile up on top of each other to the point that the family becomes dysfunctional and incapable of caring for anybody!

When serious crises occur in families, they know it and feel it, but the family members may be so overwhelmed by the experience that they do destructive things or make impulsive decisions that only make things worse. As a result tensions and problems escalate, arguments become more explosive, and family members are effectively polarized and are unable or unwilling to work together.

When things get dangerously out of control, bad things usually happen. These negative outcomes may occur in every aspect of life. As the primary caregiver you may develop mental and physical health problems that not only cause pain and suffering but incapacitate you as an effective caregiver. Your work productivity may be affected, and your boss and co-workers may not be sympathetic. Your friends may seem to desert you. They in turn may feel rebuffed by you, unable to tolerate your persistent anger, depression, or unpleasant behavior.

Bad things may also happen to your family. Tension may appear in myriad ways. Young children may begin to act out at home or school. You and other family members may be so busy fighting with each other that your parents' needs are neglected. Furthermore, the energy invested in fighting becomes all-consuming and ruins the quality of life for everyone.

Violence, abuse, and neglect of parents are other possible outcomes. Indeed, serious physical abuse—kicking, hitting, punching, threatening, or using a weapon are common experiences in about 20 percent of families that are caring for a chronically ill parent. Sometimes family members hurt their parents and sometimes the parents seriously injure the caregiver. And sometimes both parties hurt each other.

You can reduce your risk of losing control and getting into these serious difficulties. It is important to recognize the signs when you or your family, including young children, are vulnerable or in trouble and to get help. This chapter describes ways you can evaluate your risks and includes several exercises by which you can evaluate how well you are taking care of yourself, how you feel about yourself, what types of other life changes and stresses are piling up on you, how well you are coping, and how burdened you feel by the caregiving. These exercises are included to help you identify your level of distress and motivate you to think about what you can do to reduce your vulnerability.

STRATEGIES FOR STAYING IN CONTROL

Three basic strategies can help you prevent serious crises and re-duce your vulnerability to losing control. The first is to understand your attitudes and beliefs about how much control you should have over what happens to your parents as well as what you can do for them. The second relates to how you use a social support system—the people who can help you, usually your family and friends but also your boss and work associates, health care and community care providers, and other people in your neighborhood or com-munity. The third strategy involves improving your self-esteem, or how you feel about yourself.

Understand Your Attitudes, Beliefs, and Expectations

Your concept of your ability to help your parents has a great impact on how vulnerable you are to getting into trouble. Although there is a great deal you can do for your parents, there are always limits. You can listen, be responsive to their pain or discomfort, find a good doctor or arrange for in-home help, and do many other things for them. It is important to remember that the chronic diseases of later life are by definition incurable and usually progressive. In many instances, no matter how much you do, your parents will not be cured, and over time they will get worse.

In the world of caregiving, you need to develop a different way of thinking. Let yourself be guided by a tempered optimism—be prepared to accept failure while you are trying to succeed. To as-sume that you can change the inexorable course of events "if you could only do enough" is simply wrong. It dooms you to failure and disappointment and hurts your ability to be helpful. Accept that caregiving is actually an impossible task, but by making a plan and accomplishing specific goals that are within your capabilities and financial resources, you can make important contributions to it.

Tempered optimism also means feeling good about doing your best. More than two-thirds of caregivers report that they are satis-fied with the care they are giving to older relatives, but they also report feeling guilty that they should be doing more. Perhaps one of the most important principles of caregiving is to come to grips with the obvious—that life is finite and our economic and time resources are also finite. Just do your best, and learn to feel satisfied with that. Take things in stride, even when you fail. Feel satisfied with what you have done rather than dwell on unresolved problems, and be prepared to keep trying!

Use Your Social Support System

Caregiving is not a private matter that you must deal with alone. The chances of your developing serious health problems, losing perspective on your situation, getting fired from your job, or even committing abusive and violent acts are significantly increased when you try to go it by yourself.

Having a social support system and using it are essential for successful coping over the long haul. Your family and friends can help you create a buffer to cushion you or protect you from the stress of caregiving. They can also help you find different ways to deal with your stress.

How does your social support system help you? There are many ways. First, your family and friends are a source of comfort. They can help you feel loved and cared for at times when you feel inadequate or do not like yourself very much. Second, they can make you feel that you are doing the best you can and that you have made valuable contributions to your parents' welfare, when you may feel you have not done enough. Third, your social support network can reinforce that you belong, that you are part of a group where people have mutual obligations toward one another. Fourth, there is someone to turn to for help in an emergency, to give advice, act as a sounding board, and help with a chore at a given time.

The following three self-assessment exercises will help you focus on who is in your support system and how you have relied or not relied on them.

Exercise 1. Make a list of people whom you consider the most important in your life. Then ask yourself these questions about each of those people:

1. What are the qualities I most admire and enjoy in that person?
2. What are the qualities that person most admires and enjoys about me?
3. How frequently do I call or initiate a visit with that person?
4. How frequently do they call or initiate a visit with me?
5. How frequently do I attend church, clubs, or organizations with that person?
6. How frequently do I spend time with that person in pleasurable activities, such as going to movies and restaurants or on trips?

These questions should provoke you to think about how you relate to other people and how they relate to you. The next two self-assessment exercises are much more specific about how people do or do not assist you with caregiving. The questions were developed by Linda George, a sociologist who has specialized in understanding caregiving and social networks.

ASSESSMENT OF FAMILY NETWORK

Type of Help	*How Often You Received This Help*				
In the past year, how often did your family:	**Never**	**Rarely**	**Only when asked**	**Sometimes**	**Often**
Help you out when you were sick?	1	2	3	4	5
Shop or run errands for you?	1	2	3	4	5
Help you out with money or bills?	1	2	3	4	5
Fix things around your house?	1	2	3	4	5

Keep house for you or do household chores?	1	2	3	4	5
Give you advice on business or finances?	1	2	3	4	5
Provide companion-ship for you?	1	2	3	4	5
Give you advice on dealing with problems?	1	2	3	4	5
Provide transporta-tion for you?	1	2	3	4	5
Prepare or provide meals?	1	2	3	4	5
Stay with your parents while you were away?	1	2	3	4	5
Provide grooming services for your parents?	1	2	3	4	5

ASSESSMENT OF SOCIAL SUPPORT

Type of Help	*How Often You Received This Help*				
In the past year, how often were you able to get a friend or neighbor to:	**Never**	**Rarely**	**Only when asked**	**Sometimes**	**Often**
Help you out when you were sick?	1	2	3	4	5
Shop or run errands for you?	1	2	3	4	5
Help you out with money or bills?	1	2	3	4	5

Fix things around your house?	1	2	3	4	5
Keep house for you or do household chores?	1	2	3	4	5
Give you advice on business or finances?	1	2	3	4	5
Provide companion-ship for you?	1	2	3	4	5
Give you advice on dealing with problems?	1	2	3	4	5
Provide transporta-tion for you?	1	2	3	4	5
Prepare or provide meals?	1	2	3	4	5
Stay with your parents while you were away?	1	2	3	4	5
Provide grooming services for your parents?	1	2	3	4	5

The literature on the science of caregiving shows that among families who cope with caregiving, those with strong social support networks do better than those without such support systems. If you do not have a good support system, this is the time to reach out to a physician, clergyman, or someone you trust. It may also be appropriate to call a family meeting and discuss the situation.

Improve Your Self-Esteem

Your self-esteem is how you think and feel about yourself. Your self-esteem can be positive (I'm pretty, I'm smart, or I'm fun to be with) or it can be negative (I'm ugly, I'm stupid, or I'm afraid to fail). The more positive feelings you have about yourself, the higher your self-esteem, while the more negative thoughts you have, the lower your self-esteem.

Your self-esteem affects how you think, act, and feel about yourself and others and how successful you are in caring for yourself and others. High self-esteem can make you feel lovable, competent, effective, and productive, while low self-esteem can make you feel unloved, incompetent, ineffective, and worthless.

Feeling good about yourself is protective. It helps prevent you from spinning out of control from the challenges of parent-caring. Feeling good about yourself allows you to accept challenges, maintain your self-confidence even when you fail, and remain flexible.

How do you feel about yourself? Evaluate your level of self-esteem by honestly using the following questions. (They were developed by the Wien Center, a joint program of the Mount Sinai Medical Center and the University of Miami School of Medicine.) Most people feel bad about themselves at some time. When you answer these ten questions, think about how you feel most of the time.

1.	Are you easily hurt by criticism?	Yes	No
2.	Are you very shy or overly aggressive?	Yes	No
3.	Do you try to hide your feelings from others?	Yes	No
4.	Do you fear close relationships?	Yes	No
5.	Do you try to blame your mistakes on others?	Yes	No
6.	Do you find excuses for refusing to change?	Yes	No
7.	Do you avoid new experiences?	Yes	No
8.	Do you continuously wish you could change your physical appearance?	Yes	No
9.	Are you too modest about personal success?	Yes	No
10.	Are you glad when others fail?	Yes	No

If you answered most of these questions yes, your self-esteem probably needs improvement. Now answer the following ten questions as honestly as you can.

1.	Do you accept constructive criticism?	Yes	No
2.	Are you at ease meeting new people?	Yes	No
3.	Are you honest and open about your feelings?	Yes	No
4.	Do you value your closest relationships?	Yes	No
5.	Are you able to laugh at and learn from your own mistakes?	Yes	No
6.	Do you notice and accept changes in yourself as they occur?	Yes	No
7.	Do you look for and tackle new challenges?	Yes	No
8.	Are you confident about your physical appearance?	Yes	No
9.	Do you give yourself credit when credit is due?	Yes	No
10.	Are you happy for others when they succeed?	Yes	No

Now, if you answered yes to most of these questions, then you probably have a healthy opinion of yourself.

Tips to improve your self-esteem. You need to find time for yourself, as discussed in the last chapter. Accept your strengths and weaknesses. Everyone has them! Take time out regularly to be alone with yourself. Trust your gut reactions. Pay attention to your thoughts and feelings, and do what you think is right. Respect yourself, be proud of who you are, and approve your talents. Praise yourself. Take time to enjoy your activities.

High self-esteem does not guarantee you success with caregiving, but it does guarantee feeling good about yourself if things get rough. It is not easy to raise your self-esteem when it is low. It means taking a very hard look at yourself and changing what you do not like.

How to Recognize Whether You Are Taking Care of Yourself

Since you and other family members are the first line of defense for your parents, you need to take care of yourself. Evaluate regularly the physical, mental, and spiritual dimensions of your life. Without attending to them you risk losing control and getting into trouble!

The physical dimension includes caring for your body—getting regular exercise, eating correctly, getting enough rest. The mental dimension means keeping your mind active and finding ways to continue to educate yourself by reading and writing and doing things. The spiritual dimension is a very private one that refers to what inspires you, gives you peace of mind, and renews your internal strength. These activities can include prayer, listening to music, meditation, walks, or alone time.

Read the following statements and circle the number that indicates how well you perform each of the five areas.

	Very poor	Poor	Fair	Good	Very good
1. I exercise regularly.	1	2	3	4	5
2. I take care of my physical health.	1	2	3	4	5
3. I take time to find meaning and value in my life.	1	2	3	4	5
4. I take time to read, write, and learn new things.	1	2	3	4	5
5. I try to improve my relationships with others.	1	2	3	4	5

Total your points and divide by five to get your score. The higher your score, the more you are in control of yourself. If your score is lower than you would like it, decide what you are going to do to balance your physical, mental, and spiritual selves.

If you need to work at balancing your personal needs, this next exercise will help you redefine and reschedule personal time: Buy a small pocket calendar or diary. For the next week write down each day what you do to care for your physical, mental, and spiritual self. Be specific about the time and what you did for yourself, not for your parents or anyone else—for you only! At the end of the week, review what you have done—or not done. If you are not satisfied, keep the calendar for the next several weeks as a way of monitoring yourself. It is easy to say you are going to eat better, get enough sleep, or take time to "smell the roses." It is easy to think about doing these things but never take action. Writing is a way of holding yourself accountable. Remember, your goal is not to change your overall lifestyle. It is to get you to focus on and care for yourself.

HEALTH BEHAVIOR PROFILE
FOR EXERCISE

Exercise can be easy for some people and an anathema to others. It is extremely important for overall physical and mental fitness and is an effective remedy to vent frustrations. The following exercise profile can help you determine the adequacy of your current exercise program. It allows you to rate yourself and perhaps get ideas for what you can do to exercise if you have been neglecting it. (It was created by Phillip Rice, the author of *Stress and Health*.)

Add up all the numbers you have circled. Then count those items with a value of 1 or more, and divide that number into your total. If the result is 3 or greater, you have an excellent rating. If the result ranges between 1.5 and 3.0, you have a good exercise routine. If the result is below 1.5, you are at risk.

SELF-ASSESSMENT FOR EXERCISE

This profile will help you determine the adequacy of your current physical activities and/or exercise program. Circle the level of your participation in the listed activities.

How often do you participate in:	Never or almost never	Once a month	Once a week	2 or 3 times a week	4 or more times a week
1. Swimming	0	1	2	3	4
2. Walking (at least 1 mile)	0	1	2	3	4
3. Hiking or backpacking	0	1	2	3	4
4. Gardening	0	1	2	3	4
5. Bicycling	0	1	2	3	4
6. Calisthenics, aerobics, dance	0	1	2	3	4
7. Racquetball, tennis	0	1	2	3	4
8. Canoeing or boating	0	1	2	3	4
9. Water-skiing	0	1	2	3	4
10. Snow-skiing	0	1	2	3	4
11. Golf	0	1	2	3	4
12. Team sports	0	1	2	3	4
13. Running	0	1	2	3	4
14. Weightlifting	0	1	2	3	4
15. Other physical exercise	0	1	2	3	4

HEALTH BEHAVIOR PROFILE FOR DIET AND NUTRITION

Poor diet and nutritional habits put you at risk for many preventable problems. If you do not eat properly, you will be tired, edgy, irritable, and less effective. If your poor diet and nutritional habits are of long standing, you are probably at risk for malnutrition.

The next exercise, also developed by Phillip Rice, is not a comprehensive nutritional assessment, but is intended to help you focus on nutrition to see where you can take better care of yourself.

SELF-ASSESSMENT FOR NUTRITION AND DIET

This scale will help you compare your dietary habits with what is considered good practice. Circle the answer that most accurately describes your eating habits.

How often do you:	Once a month or less	A few times a month	Once a week	Every day
1. Not eat fruits, vegetables, fiber?	1	2	3	4
2. Drink five or more cups of coffee in a day?	1	2	3	4
3. Eat fats, red meats, dairy products?	1	2	3	4
4. Drink five or more soft drinks (diet or regular)?	1	2	3	4
5. Eat candies, sugars, pastries?	1	2	3	4
6. Take vitamin supplements?	1	2	3	4
7. Overeat at meals?	1	2	3	4
8. Eat between meals?	1	2	3	4
9. Eat while watching TV, reading, and so on?	1	2	3	4
10. Skip breakfast?	1	2	3	4
11. Skip lunch?	1	2	3	4
12. Skip dinner?	1	2	3	4
13. Use flash diets to lose weight?	1	2	3	4

| 14. | Take diet pills? | 1 | 2 | 3 | 4 |
| 15. | Use amphetamines to lose weight? | 1 | 2 | 3 | 4 |

Add up the numbers you have circled for the fifteen questions. A score lower than 20 indicates that your eating habits are excellent. A score ranging from 20 to 35 suggests good habits. A score greater than 40 suggests that you are at risk. If you scored in the high-risk zone, identify the items on the list for which you circled a 3 or a 4; these are the eating habits you need to change.

Assess Your Caregiver Burden

Caregiver burden consists of the problems experienced because of caregiving. It reflects how your personal life is constrained or limited by your caregiving activities, in your view, as well as how your parents' behavior disrupts your relationship with them and others.

Burden is something that almost every caregiver reports. It is normal to feel burdened by the responsibilities—burden is a complex factor. The burden you feel is a function of how much you have to do, how much caregiving distresses you, how effective you are in coping, the effectiveness of your social support system, your own health and expectations, and other life stresses, as well as your personality style.

The items below, developed by Stephanie McFall, should help you assess how burdened you are. Answer each of the following yes or no.

1. I have to take care of my parent(s) when I don't feel well enough.

2. Taking care of my parent(s) is hard on me emotionally.

3. Taking care of my parent(s) limits my social life or free time.

4. Taking care of my parent(s) has caused my health to get worse.

5. Care costs more than I can really afford.

6. I have to give my parent(s) almost constant attention.

7. Sometimes my parent(s) forgets things, gets confused, or refuses to cooperate.

8. Sometimes my parent(s) embarrasses me or others.

9. Sometimes my parent(s) lapses into periods of memory loss.

10. Sometimes my parent(s) becomes upset and yells at me.

Give yourself 1 point for every yes you answered; each point represents a problem. If you identified 1–3 problems, you are experiencing mild burden, 4–6 problems means moderate burden, and 7–10 is severe burden.

A high score does not mean that you are necessarily in danger of bad health or losing control. You should regard your score as just one way to examine the stress and strain you are under. You also need to think about your sense of burden in relation to other feelings, such as your caregiver satisfaction.

It is possible to feel burdened and also satisfied with your caregiving. Rate how often you have had the following sentiments:

		Never	Rarely	Half the time	More frequently than half	Nearly always
1.	Helping my parent(s) makes me feel closer to them.	1	2	3	4	5
2.	I enjoy being with my parent(s).	1	2	3	4	5
3.	Taking responsibility for my parent(s) gives me a sense of self-esteem.	1	2	3	4	5
4.	My parent(s) show real appreciation for what I do.	1	2	3	4	5
5.	My parent's(s') pleasure gives me pleasure.	1	2	3	4	5

Add up your scores. The lower your score, the more negative you feel; the higher your score, the more satisfied you are. A high burden score coupled with a low satisfaction score is an indicator that you would benefit from talking with someone to get some emotional assistance or support.

WARNING SIGNS THAT YOUNG CHILDREN ARE AT RISK

Children, even young children where appropriate, can be valuable partners in family caregiving. Children are full of thoughts and feelings about what is going on. They have a legitimate right, like everyone else in the family, to be kept informed, to be allowed to express their feelings, and to be involved in ways with which they are comfortable. Involving children also creates opportunities for their parents to spend time with them and teach them the value of caring for others.

To exclude children often creates a number of problems, including anxiety from not knowing what is wrong, guilt that they are somehow responsible, or anger that they are being excluded. The following are some of the warning signs that your child may not be coping well with the stresses of caregiving in your household.

- The appearance of new and strange fears, such as fear of the dark, of strangers, of being alone or sleeping alone

- Insistence on having mother or father nearby and refusing to go to previously favorite places

- Significant change in emotions such as crying, sleep disturbances with nightmares, irritability, or withdrawal from friends

- Sudden changes in school performance

The most important clues are marked changes in a child's usual behaviors. If you are concerned that your children are being affected adversely, it is important to spend time with them to talk the issues through. There are a number of children's books that may be useful for you to read together as a way of developing a discussion (see Selected Readings). It is also important to talk with teachers if your child is getting into trouble or doing poorly.

A Look at Work Stress

Caregiving can have a significant impact on you and your work performance. A number of studies have shown that 20 to 30 percent of caregivers take significant time off and another 20 to 30 percent quit their jobs. Furthermore, the stress associated with caregiving can spill over into the workplace. Behavioral symptoms of work stress include lowered productivity, avoidance of work and procrastination, increased hostility with the boss or co-workers, job dissatisfaction, increased fatigue, job burnout, and increased sick days.

If you are working outside the home, answer the questions in the following self-assessment of work changes.

ASSESSMENT OF WORK CHANGES

1. How many hours do you work outside the home?
2. Have you had to adjust your work schedule to care for your parents?
   a. Yes, cut back hours
   b. Yes, took time off
   c. Yes, quit work
   d. No changes

Answer yes or no to the following:

3. Have you thought about quitting work to care for your parents?
4. Have you ever felt that your parents would be better off if you quit work?
5. Have you discussed quitting work with family members or others?
6. Have you discussed quitting work with your parents?
7. Is it likely that you will quit work to care for your parents in the near future?

There is no total score for this exercise. The questions are presented to help you examine how close you may be to making the decision to quit work. If you are unhappy and concerned about your ability to keep working but you want to or must work to support your family, talk with your employer or someone in the employee assistance program in your company. Today, more than twenty-four hundred companies, including many of the *Fortune* 500, have private employee assistance programs that offer a wide variety of workshops and courses to help you deal with work problems, including caring for the needs of aging parents and relatives. These can include personal counseling, stress management classes, job retraining, career counseling, child-care programs, and health care and nutrition programs.

THE PILEUP OF LIFE STRESSES

Caregiving may be a potential stress for you and your family, but other life changes are also likely to take their toll on you as well. The research of Thomas Holmes of the University of Washington and Richard Rahe of the U.S. Navy Medical Neuropsychiatric Research Unit led to a better understanding of what life-change situations are most stressful and are associated with a risk for health problems. They developed the Social Readjustment Rating Scale, which is reproduced below.

Go through the items on the scale and circle the number on the left representing any events or conditions you have experienced in the last six months. Then, for each such event, circle the life-change unit on the right.

Rank	Life Event	LCU (Life-Change Unit)
1	Death of a spouse	100
2	Divorce	73
3	Marital separation	65

4	Jail term	63
5	Death of close family member	63
6	Personal injury or illness	53
7	Marriage	50
8	Being fired at work	47
9	Marital reconciliation	45
10	Retirement	45
11	Change in health of parent	44
12	Pregnancy	40
13	Sexual difficulties	39
14	Gain of new family member	39
15	Business readjustment	39
16	Change in financial state	38
17	Death of close friend	37
18	Change to different line of work	36
19	Change in number of arguments with spouse	35
20	Mortgage of more than $100,000	31
21	Foreclosure of mortgage or loan	30
22	Change in responsibilities at work	29
23	Child's leaving home	29
24	Trouble with in-laws	29
25	Outstanding personal achievement	28
26	Spouse's beginning or stopping work	26
27	Beginning or completing school	26
28	Change in living conditions	25
29	Revision of personal habits	24
30	Trouble with boss	23
31	Change in work hours or conditions	20
32	Change in residence	20
33	Change in school	20
34	Change in recreation	19
35	Change in church activities	19

36	Change in social activities	18
37	Mortgage or loan of less than $100,000	17
38	Change in sleeping habits	16
39	Change in number of family get-togethers	15
40	Change in eating habits	13
41	Vacation	13
42	Christmas	12
43	Minor violations of the law	11

Add up the life-change units you have circled. Your total score is a summation of your life changes—both good and bad—over the past six months. A total of 150–199 LCUs defines a mild life crisis, 200–299 LCUs a moderate life crisis, and anything above 300 a major life crisis. A very high score indicates that you may be at risk for health problems. While not everyone with a high score gets sick, if your score is high, it may be useful to talk with friends or professionals.

EXAMINE YOUR COPING STYLES

Caregiving is a major ongoing life event that requires active coping. The large scientific literature on coping with stress shows that people have many different coping styles. *Coping* is defined as any emotional, cognitive, or behavioral response to reduce, prevent, or eliminate stress. Examples of emotional coping are getting angry or bitter, feeling sad and depressed, or feeling anxious and upset. *Cognitive coping* refers to a range of responses such as accepting the situation, setting up goals to deal with the problems, coming up with different solutions, denying or suppressing any thoughts, and turning to religion or prayer. Behavioral or problem-solving responses may include looking for relevant information, seeking emotional support or joining a support group, or changing something about yourself to be able to deal with the situation more successfully.

To find out what coping styles you use, perform this self-assessment. Answer yes or no to each of the following:

I have accepted the situation.

I refuse to let it get to me.

I have made the best of it.

I waited for the problem to work itself out.

If you answered any of these items yes, you are using a coping style known as acceptance. It is helpful to accept what is happening to you. You may not be able to change what is happening to your parents, but you can accept the reality.

Now answer these eight items, again with yes or no:

I get upset and depressed.

I became angry, bitter, and resentful.

I prepared for the worst.

I tried to see the positive side of the situation.

I kept my feelings to myself.

I tried to reduce my tension by eating/drinking.

I tried to reduce my tension by smoking more.

I tried to reduce my tension by exercising more.

If you answered yes to any of these statements, you are using emotion-focused coping strategies.

Go on to the next nine items, again answering yes or no:

I felt inspired to be creative in solving the problem.

I came up with a couple of different solutions to the problem.

I changed something about myself so I could deal with the situation better.

I did something totally new to solve the problem.

I read books, newspapers, and/or magazine articles to learn how to deal with the problem.

I drew on my past experience.

I took things one day at a time.

I talked with a professional person about the situation.

I spoke with my spouse or other relative about the situation.

If you answered yes to any of these, you are using problem-solving strategies.

Now respond to the last two items:

I turned to religion or prayer.

I hoped a miracle would happen.

A yes to either of these indicates that you are using intrapsychic or spiritual coping styles.

There is no score in this exercise. Its purpose is to help you identify and clarify the coping styles you use. Most people activate several different coping styles, and they find that some are more effective than others. Doing something about your situation, setting goals, looking for information, and getting emotional support and reassurance from others are generally effective over the long term, even if you do not have immediate success with them.

Not only can persistent emotional responses lead to a negative psychological state, but they can keep you from doing anything to alleviate your stress, express your feelings, and modify your situation. If you have just moved your father or mother into a nursing home, for example, it is normal to cope by feeling many emotions—anger, guilt, sadness. But to continue to feel these negative emotions without adopting cognitive and behavioral coping strategies to accept what had to be done has a high likelihood of affecting your health. There is evidence that more than a third of caregivers continue to feel significant stress after institutionalizing a relative and continue to use poor coping strategies. A significant percentage use drugs for their nerves, drink excessively, and continue to feel depressed and guilty. To continue to feel anger, depression, and anxiety for a long time is dangerous to your health!

LOSING CONTROL

The following story is not an unusual or complicated family situation. It illustrates the dire trouble people can get into when they lose control. These situations are preventable!

Doris Gordon invited her elderly father, Bob, to live with her after her mother died. Six months later, he began to have some dizzy spells and progressive memory problems, and the doctors finally diagnosed him as suffering from Alzheimer's disease.

Doris found it more and more difficult to deal with her father as his health worsened. Just to get him up in the morning, feed him, and dress him usually took three hours or more. She felt boxed in by the pressures of doing everything, but getting help was out of the question. Taking care of him alone while maintaining her real estate business was what she expected of herself. After all, she had nursed her husband for the four years before he died, and she would do no less for her father.

Doris had three daughters—Julie, Ellery, and Alice—but she did not want to burden them by asking them to help her. The two older ones, Julie and Ellery, had careers and families of their own. Her youngest, Alice, had schizophrenia and had been a source of great upset over the years. Alice had her own apartment and a job as a checkout clerk, but Doris still gave her a monthly allowance for rent and food.

Bob began to have violent outbursts almost daily. He even hurt Doris on more than one occasion. Doris became afraid, and she used restraints to deal with him for several months. She would handcuff or tie him to the bedpost while he napped in the late morning. This would allow her to leave him for several hours and go out to deal with her real estate clients.

The future looked bleak for Doris. She had never dreamed she would have serious financial problems. Her real estate business was successful, but it was not enough to meet her financial needs over the long term. Doris was scared for the first time in her life. This fear of the future, coupled with her father's unpredictable rages and client pressures, all worked together to push Doris over the edge, to the point that she abused her father.

The Hurtful Consequences of Losing Control

This upsetting story is only one example of what can happen when family life is disrupted by the pileup of life stresses. Serious problems usually emerge when stressors are hurtful, they last a long time and overwhelm your ability to cope. Serious stress may not only lead to negligence or violence, it may intensify other family problems.

Caregivers are at high risk for serious mental health problems that may cause them to harm others—even caregivers like Doris Gordon, who have weathered crises in the past. Unfortunately, other family members frequently do not recognize that something is wrong, and the "abuser" usually feels too ashamed or afraid to ask for help. Ellery and Julie had always seen their mother as a tireless, strong-willed, and capable woman, and they did not recognize it as a cry for help when Doris began calling them several times a day. Doris repeated herself in telling them how well she was doing and the daughters missed this signal that all was not well.

There are different forms of abuse—physical, material, and neglect. Physical abuse is the deliberate infliction of physical pain, injury, or unreasonable restraint. Material abuse is the misuse of a relative's property, money, or other assets. It may include willful deception about finances, mismanagement of funds, taking money, or diversion of income. Neglect is the deprivation of a relative of appropriate food, clothing, shelter, or health care, creating a danger to health.

Fortunately, we are beginning to learn what causes these destructive interactions as well as what can be done to prevent them. Physical abuse and neglect are in fact the common results of the severe and unrelenting stress associated with the ongoing responsibility for a disabled chronically ill relative. They are particularly likely to occur when the caregiver is depressed or is not getting help and support from other family members or from clergy or service agencies. And this is precisely where the problem lies. Usually caregivers believe they can do everything themselves and they refuse help, or else others are unaware of the seriousness of the situation. Doris, for example, believed that she could "go it alone" and would not ask for help.

Eventually, Doris followed her minister's recommendation that she see a psychiatrist. The psychiatrist diagnosed her with a clinical depression and recommended a combination of antidepressant medication and psychotherapy. In one sense Doris was relieved to know that she had a psychiatric illness because it explained why she had hurt her father the way she did. She was also embarrassed and afraid that family and friends would not understand. The psychiatrist asked Doris to invite her daughters to a session so he could explain to them what had happened and why and involve them in making plans for the future. Doris could not continue to go it alone. She had to find ways to let her daughters help her.

Although there is no right way to care for someone, there are some wrong ways. One of them is to do everything alone and hide your needs from others, for whatever reason. The result can be disastrous, as it was for Doris, who developed a clinical depression and then spun out of control into a violent relationship with her father. How did the violence evolve?

After her father got sick, Doris lived by two simple rules: First: "Keep working!" Second: "You can do everything yourself!" And the sicker her dad became, the more Doris clung to her usual patterns. Damn the torpedoes and full steam ahead! She willed herself to care for him, to see clients, and to make it through each day. But ultimately her strong will disabled her. Doris concentrated so hard on her narrow rules that she became willfully blind to what was happening. She allowed no one to get close enough to her to give her another point of view, and her will to keep going became all she had. No human being can resolve their life problems through sheer willpower.

What to Do When Things Are Really out of Control

When you are in trouble, get help! Whether you see a counselor or a friend, you need others around you to get a handle on what is happening. Refer to Chapter 3—there is nothing wrong with seeking out professional help. This may be the quickest way for you to regain control of your life. Do not insist that you can do it alone. You may not be able to free yourself from your burdens without the help of others.

Do not let yourself suffer from a false sense that you are in control. You may truly believe that you are handling the situation as well as anyone can. This belief may be absolutely correct, or it might be an illusion.

There is a story about a prisoner who is tied up and thrown into a deep pit. After a great struggle, the prisoner escapes from the ropes and yells, "I'm free! I'm free!" The prisoner is certainly *more* free, since he is able to move around. But his freedom is an illusion. He is still at the bottom of the pit. In order to get out of the pit, he needs not only freedom from his bonds but help getting out of the pit.

As discussed throughout this book, caring involves knowing yourself and how to care for yourself, much as athletes know their physical ability and train themselves to maintain and enhance that ability. Understanding your family and their needs as well as the needs of your parents and all the resources that are available is another crucial set of factors that you have to manage, and understanding the seriousness of the problem and specifically what help is required is yet another necessity.

But sometimes there is nothing that can help or make any major difference in the outcome. Not all problems are solvable. We all accept that taxes and death are inevitable, but how we deal with them can affect us deeply.

After struggling to provide care, we may eventually come face-to-face with the possibility that nothing more can be done. Death may be a release for some but a tragedy in the eyes of others. The process of caring for a dying person whom you love—or are bonded to—can be excruciating. The next chapter takes you into that process with the hope that it will help you deal with death—the inevitable fact of life.

7

LETTING GO AND MOVING ON

Letting go and moving on may be the most difficult aspect of caregiving because it is about coming to terms with your parents and yourself. There are no simple prescriptions for how to do this because everyone is different. There are, however, some useful books with which you can reflect upon your experience and perhaps develop some closure or understanding about what has happened. Ralph Keyes's anthology *Sons on Fathers* beautifully expresses the powerful and changing relationship of fathers and sons throughout the life cycle. We mention it here because the theme of the book is the theme of this chapter—as Keyes puts it, "Reconciliation may not always be possible. Understanding is."

THE SEVEN PHASES OF MOVING ON

There are at least seven phases in letting go and moving on. The first three are actually issues to be dealt with early in the caregiving process; the last four are issues for later. The seven phases are as follows:

1. Let go of the belief that you direct your parents' lives.

2. Set limits on what you do.

3. Let others help.

4. Develop some compassionate distance to your parents as they deteriorate.

5. Let your parents move into supportive housing or a nursing home, if necessary.

6. Prepare for dying and death.

7. Move on.

In one sense, letting go actually begins at the very time you get started caregiving and define your role in it. This first phase of letting go is confronting what your job is in the context of the reality of the situation. As we have seen, your role is to care, not to direct or manipulate the lives of other people as you think best. A helpful rule of thumb is the golden rule—to do for your parents as you would want done to you. There is also another version of the golden rule: Do not do to others what you would not want done to yourself.

The second phase is the realization that while there are many things you can do to help your parents, there are limits. You need to curb any belief that you can rescue them from the inevitable progression of a chronic illness, but maintain a focus on doing what can be reasonably done to help them without losing hope for today. There are times, particularly when your parents are close to death, where you can do little but be there. And this is important! Conveying support, giving affection, and touching to ease pain and loneliness are powerful gifts from one human being to another.

The third phase is letting others help your parents. As discussed earlier, this can mean permitting home aides, chore workers, and nurses to come into the house, or it can mean enrolling your parents in day care or respite care programs in the community. Finding good providers can mean the difference between helping your parents continue to live at home instead of going into a nursing home. There is also evidence that many older people prefer paid help to family members for assistance in personal care activities. For the person in need, this preserves their dignity and place within the family and reduces their guilt over burdening people they love.

The fourth challenge is learning skills to modulate being close to your parents while achieving some distance. A paradox of family life is that it encourages members to be interdependent and independent at the same time. A number of family therapists have described family membership as a special belonging that gives people both roots and wings. This seeming conflict is played out in all aspects of family life, but when parents are aging and frail, it is essential to come to terms in explicit ways with how to be compassionate without being so overwhelmed that you lose your ability to make sensible decisions. Letting go or pulling away from them at times does not mean that you do not care for them. On the contrary, it means that you know how to find the appropriate emotional distance to protect both them and yourself in order to care for them and everyone else.

Becoming too close can smother and infantilize your parent. Not only does this behavior not help your parent, it makes it far more difficult for you to handle problems that need mature judgment. On the other hand, keeping too great a distance brings other problems. The challenge is to recognize that the appropriate emotional spacing is needed and that regulating emotional closeness and distance is a dynamic, changing process.

A fifth phase for some families is having to find a more supportive living arrangement or a nursing home. This phase can be traumatic because it is often a last resort, occurring after the family has exhausted its personal and financial resources. The sad irony is that even after the goal of living at home has been achieved for long years, caring may still end in institutionalization. Unfortunately, nursing home placement usually occurs with guilt, anger, and upset—many see it as constituting failure.

Institutional care should be considered a technical rather than a moral issue. Although families can provide care and support, they should recognize that the need may exceed their capacity. It is not a failure to hospitalize your parents for certain medical procedures that cannot be done as outpatient or one-day surgicare. By the same token, if your parents need a level of nursing care that your family cannot provide, a more structured supportive environment becomes an important option. The mistake is to believe that such care is bad, to omit thinking through the issues of institutional care, to omit examining what is available, and then to get caught in a crisis having to settle for a suboptimal environment—and feel guilty.

The sixth issue in letting go is what happens to everyone—death. It can be rapid, or it can be prolonged with pain and suffering when parents die slowly. The simple, irrevocable reality of life is that each of us is going to die. Therefore, one of the best things you can do is be prepared for it. Talk about it with your parents and others in the family, and have a plan of action written down for both them and you. This plan should cover such basic issues as funeral arrangements, burial, and legacies. Each of us needs our survivors to carry out our wishes, and we owe them whatever help we can give them in doing so. Terrible family disputes concerning each issue involved in dying can and should be avoided by discussions. It is realistic and important to come to grips with decisions so that everyone will know what your parents want to happen to them. Issues ranging from autopsies to who gets family heirlooms are charged and are ideally settled before death occurs.

The final phase comes after death, and it involves integrating all that has happened and moving on with your life. A number of books have been written that record what Louis Begley called the "humiliation and torture that old age and medical science inflict on parents." But many other books are testimony to the beauty of the human spirit. Some of the best are Philip Roth's *Patrimony*, Simone de Beauvoir's *A Very Easy Death*, and Andrew Malcolm's *Someday*. These and others listed at the back of this book may be painful reading in one sense, but they are also more. They record how each writer came to have a richer understanding of their parents and their family.

Caregiving takes you through an extensive grieving and healing process. Restructuring your life and moving on is the last part of that process. It takes not only a deliberate effort but patience and acceptance to let time heal you. There is a story about a very old king who had grown tired of fighting the emotional battles of growing old. For his hundredth birthday he let it be known throughout his kingdom that he wanted something that could make him happy when he was sad and sad when he felt happy. A very wise man brought him a ring he had made with a single inscription: This too shall pass.

1. Let go of the belief that you direct your parents' lives.

You may be an adviser to your parents and sometimes an advocate for their well-being. You may even hold fiscal authority or the right to obtain or refuse medical care for them. You do not control them, however. They have the right to make decisions about their own health, lifestyle, body, and property—and to have such decisions carried out as they wish. It is not your role to make decisions for them but where possible to help them get information, clarify their options, understand the consequences of different options, and figure out what values and beliefs are motivating their decisions. While you cannot direct them, you can do things that promote their overall health and well-being. Sometimes you will disagree with a decision they make. At such times you should take special care to understand them and their needs and wishes.

Medical care is an area where you can play an important role—but again, your parents' wishes are the ones that dictate what happens. You can also make a difference in the quality of care your parents receive when they are hospitalized or move into a nursing home. Chances are that you will help make many difficult decisions, and it is the nature of medical care today that you will deal with a large cast of players—insurance agents, lawyers, hospital administrators, and many different doctors, nurses, social workers, therapists, and other professionals.

You have an important responsibility to be informed about what is going on and to help your parents be informed. Physicians are experts in medicine, and other professionals are experts in their areas, but your parents are experts at knowing what they feel, and you are an expert on your family. The best medical care decisions are made when everyone is working together. Your responsibility is to make sure your parents have the information they need to make informed decisions. This can be especially difficult when they are in a hospital and physical and mental illness impair their decision-making abilities. It is even more difficult if you and your parents have not discussed these issues beforehand. Therefore, a positive way to let go is to be proactive and empower your parents to prepare for making decisions in the future when they may not be able to communicate what they want in a hospital or nursing home setting.

It is wise to prepare yourself for difficult times if your parents are seriously injured, in a persistent confused state, or so severely cognitively impaired by dementia that they are unable to make decisions. There are two documents that you and your parents should discuss: a living will and a durable powers of attorney for health care decision making. These "advance directives" are legal tools that specify a person's preferences in advance, when they are unable to express them. People construct them when they are of sound mind, but they take effect only if they should become incapacitated. Used together or separately, a living will and a durable power of attorney will be helpful for both your parents and you. Dr. Nancy Dubler, a medical ethicist in New York, provides extensive detailed information on these two tools in her book *Ethics on Call*.

Suggest to your parents that they talk with their physician about these tools at their next office visit or checkup. Dr. Dubler lists ten questions they can ask to stimulate the discussion.

- What possible health problems do you see emerging in the future given my present state of health, my medical history, and that of my family?

- What paths might my particular condition take that could impair my ability to participate in decisions about my care? Is that likely?

- Are there some articles and books I could read about my condition?

- How do you feel about honoring any specific instructions I might leave about my care? Would you object to honoring a Do Not Resuscitate order or a directive, under some conditions, to terminate care?

- Can I appoint someone to make decisions for me? Do you know what the law and practice are in this state governing these kinds of appointments? Do you know where I can find out?

- How do my wishes get communicated to the hospital if I am hospitalized?

- Do you see your role as an advocate for my wishes?

- Would you be more comfortable following my wishes, documented in a living will, or the specific directions of my designated decider?

- How do you feel about removing respirators or feeding tubes from patients whose prognosis is hopeless?

- Would you help family members or friends reach that decision if the situation were hopeless, and I had no possibility of returning to a sapient state or of even relating to and responding to another human being?

Involving physicians and others to discuss these issues with you and your parents provides a shared basis for you to plan the future and develop a clear understanding of what your parents want under certain medical circumstances. This shared knowledge can be a source of comfort and relief because the decisions will have been made before the crisis occurs. This process allows you to let go of the anxieties caused by not being prepared to make difficult decisions.

2. Set limits on what you do.

Since the needs of any human being are virtually limitless, the needs of your parents could be overwhelming. But there are realistic limits to what you can do for them, to how many of their needs you can meet. Their needs, interests, and rights must be balanced against those of other people in the family. When your parent is in the hospital, there are clear rules for making decisions about medical care. Patients have the right of autonomy—to make decisions about their body if they have decision-making capacities, to establish advance directives in the event they are incapacitated.

Outside the hospital there are many decisions about daily living that must be made in which your parents' needs must be dealt with in relation to others. You, as the primary family caregiver, and the other family members have the right to be considered in any decisions made. Strategies to help your parents and to balance family needs to accommodate aging parents are discussed in Chapter 5. Whether your parents like it or not, they will need to accommodate their family's ability to meet their needs.

3. Let others help.

Throughout this book we have emphasized the value of a social support system as well as community services in taking some of the pressures off you. Test yourself by reading through the following list of services and check off those you have heard of and those you have been able to find and use to support your caregiving efforts.

ASSESSMENT OF COMMUNITY SERVICES

	Have you heard of it?		Have you used it?		How many times a month did you use it?
Legal services	Yes	No	Yes	No	_____
Financial aid services	Yes	No	Yes	No	_____
Meal services	Yes	No	Yes	No	_____
Home repair services	Yes	No	Yes	No	_____
Homemaker services	Yes	No	Yes	No	_____
Care services	Yes	No	Yes	No	_____
Escort services	Yes	No	Yes	No	_____
Transportation services	Yes	No	Yes	No	_____

Shopping services	Yes	No	Yes	No	_____
Friendly visitors	Yes	No	Yes	No	_____
Telephone assurance	Yes	No	Yes	No	_____
Home health care services	Yes	No	Yes	No	_____
Home attendant	Yes	No	Yes	No	_____
Day care or respite care services	Yes	No	Yes	No	_____
Family support groups	Yes	No	Yes	No	_____

If you are not aware of the various services, call your state department on aging (see Appendix B) or your local area agency on aging, located in the yellow pages.

4. Develop some compassionate distance to your parents as they deteriorate.

When people are very ill, suffering in great pain, and dying, the emotions you feel when you are with them can be overwhelming. If you let these feelings incapacitate you, it will be impossible for you to be supportive of them or to protect yourself. Physicians and other health professionals receive considerable clinical training that teaches them to be both compassionate and distant. Such professionals train with many patients under supervision, yet many still have difficulty in dealing with the emotional burden of caring.

The balance between callousness and being emotionally overwhelmed requires that you schedule time both with your parents and away from them. Make a schedule or keep a calendar to spend time with your parents, but it is just as important for you to find ways to get away by yourself or with friends, refresh yourself, and find pleasant activities to balance the hurt and anguish. If you are emotionally fragile, if you cannot focus on anything or anyone else and you cannot get away, or if you find yourself angry, unfeeling, and irritated most of the time, you may need help. Refer back to

Chapter 3 and review the material on depression. Consider finding a professional to talk with you.

5. Let your parents move into supportive housing or a nursing home, if necessary.

This can be one of the most difficult and traumatic decisions to make, especially when your parents have repeatedly told you "Don't ever put me in a nursing home" or if you have promised them you would not. Nursing homes can be a necessary alternative to keeping a relative at home. Making this decision is often a complex and upsetting process. Fortunately, Seth Goldsmith has written an excellent guide called *Choosing a Nursing Home*, and we have also written a detailed chapter on just this issue in our book *The Loss of Self: A Family Resource for Alzheimer's Disease*.

Most people do not expect that they will ever go into a nursing home, but a recent study shows that almost half of all Americans who reach sixty-five will spend some time in a nursing home. Approximately 1.5 million Americans now live in them, and in forty years, if current trends continue, it is estimated that as many as six million people could be living in such settings.

Alternatives to nursing homes include Meals on Wheels, home health care, homemakers, day care, home care, board and care, or assisted care living arrangements. These are each defined and described in Appendix A. Since the range of such services varies greatly among individual communities, we have included contacts in the appendix to help you find out what is available in your situation. In addition, most hospital social work departments can help direct you to such services. Ask your pastor or minister, priest or rabbi whom you can contact for such help.

Nursing homes are important and necessary considerations when parents are chronically ill and disabled and other resources are not available. The following brief questionnaire was developed by Richard Morcyz, a psychologist at the University of Pittsburgh, to quantify the desire to institutionalize. Answer the six questions as honestly as you can.

ASSESSMENT: DESIRE TO INSTITUTIONALIZE

Have you ever considered moving your parent into a nursing home or assisted care living facility?	No	Yes	Don't know
Have you ever felt your parent would be better off in a nursing home or boarding home?	No	Yes	Don't know
Have you ever discussed institutionalization with family members or other persons?	No	Yes	Don't know
Have you ever discussed institutionalization with your parent?	No	Yes	Don't know
Is it likely that you will move your parent into a nursing home?	No	Yes	Don't know
Have you taken steps toward placement?	No	Yes	Don't know

Give yourself one point for every item where you answered yes. If you have a score of three or higher, you should consult Goldsmith's book or others in the Selected Readings list. Put as much time and effort into selecting the right nursing home for your parent as you would a new home. That means you need to get information to make an informed decision, and you need to visit these institutions to find one you and they can live with. You will want a place that maximizes individual preferences, privacy, and choice at all times of the day and where life is regimented as little as possible.

6. Prepare for dying and death.

Create a plan. Discuss all the possibilities that could occur when your parents die, and develop a plan based upon your parents' wishes and values. The following values history form, developed by Dr. Joan McIver Gibson with Dr. Nancy Dubler, provides an effective mechanism for you and your parents to approach some difficult and painful issues. Answering these questions will help prepare you before a medical crisis occurs.

VALUES HISTORY FORM

Section 1 asks a number of questions about your attitude toward your health; feelings about doctors and nurses; thoughts about independence and control; personal relationships; your overall attitudes to life, illness, dying, and death; your religious beliefs; your living situation; feelings about finance; and even wishes concerning your funeral. There are many ways to approach these questions. You may want to write down your thoughts before talking with anyone else, or you might prefer to start by asking the important people in your life to come together and talk about you—and their answers to these questions.

Section 2 allows you to record both written and oral instructions you might already have prepared. If you have not written or talked about these issues, you may want to leave this section and come back to it when you have completed section 1.

Often these deep and intimate topics are difficult to consider and painful to talk about. The goal of the values history form is to help spur and support these conversations when it is easier to have them—before a medical crisis occurs.

As you continue to grow and change, so will your values and ideas, and so may the values reflected in the values history form. You may want to come back to this form every few years, to reconsider and reevaluate your preferences and wishes. The values history can be an important form to complete in preparation for the living will or health care proxy.

Name: _____

Date: _____

If someone assisted you in completing this form, please fill in his or her name, address, and relationship to you.

Name: _____

Address: _____

_____

Relationship: _____

The purpose of this form is to assist you in thinking about and writing down what is important to you about your health. If you should at some time become unable to make health care decisions for yourself, your thoughts as expressed on this form may help others make a decision for you in accordance with what you have chosen.

The first section of this form asks whether you have already expressed your wishes concerning medical treatment through either written or oral commitments, and if not, whether you would like to do so now. The second section of this form provides an opportunity for you to discuss your values, wishes, and preferences in a number of different areas such as your personal relationships, your overall attitude toward life, and your thoughts on illness.

SECTION 1

A.   Written Legal Documents

Have you written any of the following legal documents? If so, please complete the requested information.

LIVING WILL

Date written: _____

Document location: _____

Comments (my limitations, special requests)

_____

_____

_____

_____

DURABLE POWER OF ATTORNEY

Date written: _____

Document location: _____

Comments (whom have you named to be your decision maker?):

_____

_____

_____

_____

DURABLE POWER OF ATTORNEY FOR HEALTH CARE DECISIONS

Date written: _____

Document location: _____

Comments (whom have you named to be your decision maker?)

_____

_____

_____

_____

B. Wishes concerning specific medical procedures

If you have ever expressed your wishes, either written or orally, concerning any of the following medical procedures, please complete the requested information. If you have not previously indicated your wishes on these procedures and would like to do so now, please complete this information.

ORGAN DONATION

To whom expressed: _____

If oral, when? _____

If written, when? _____

Document location: _____

Comments: _____

KIDNEY DIALYSIS

To whom expressed: _____

If oral, when? _____

If written, when? _____

Document location: _____

Comments: _____

CARDIOPULMONARY RESUSCITATION (CPR)

To whom expressed: _____

If oral, when? _____

If written, when? _____

Document location: _____

Comments: _____

RESPIRATION

To whom expressed: _____

If oral, when? _____

If written, when? _____

Document location: _____

Comments: _____

ARTIFICIAL NUTRITION

To whom expressed: _____

If oral, when? _____

If written, when? _____

Document location: _____

Comments: _____

ARTIFICIAL HYDRATION

To whom expressed: _____

If oral, when? _____

If written, when? _____

Document location: _____

Comments: _____

C.   General Concerns

Do you wish to make any general comments about the information you provided in this section?

_____

_____

SECTION 2

A.   Your overall attitude toward your health

1. How would you describe your current health status? If you currently have any medical problems, how would you describe them?

    _____

    _____

2. If you have current medical problems, in what ways, if any, do they affect your ability to function?

_____

_____

3. How do you feel about your current health status?

_____

_____

4. How well are you able to meet the basic necessities of life—eating, food preparation, sleeping, personal hygiene, etc.?

_____

_____

5. Do you wish to make any general comments about your overall health?

_____

_____

B. Your perception of the role of your doctor and other health caregivers

1. Do you like your doctor?

_____

_____

2. Do you trust your doctor?

_____

_____

3. Do you think your doctor should make the final decisions regarding any treatment you might need?

_____

_____

4. How do you relate to your caregivers, including nurses, therapists, chaplains, social workers, etc.?

_____

_____

5. Do you wish to make any general comments about your doctors and other health professionals?

_____

_____

C. **Your thoughts about independence and control**

1. How important is independence and self-sufficiency in your life?

_____

_____

2. If you were to experience decreased physical and mental abilities, how would that affect your attitude toward independence and self-sufficiency?

_____

_____

3. Do you wish to make any general comments about the value of independence and control in your life?

_____

_____

D. **Your personal relationships**

1. Do you expect that your friends, family, and/or others support your decisions regarding medical treatment you may need now or in the future?

_____

_____

2. Have you made any arrangements for your family or friends to make medical treatment decisions on your behalf? If so, who agreed to make decisions for you and in what circumstances?

_____

_____

3. What, if any, unfinished business from the past are you concerned about (e.g., personal and family relationships, business and legal matters)?

_____

_____

4. What role do your family and friends play in your life?

_____

_____

5. Do you wish to make any general comments about the personal relationships in your life?

_____

_____

E. Your overall attitude toward life

1. What activities do you enjoy (e.g., hobbies, watching TV, etc.)?

_____

_____

2. Are you happy to be alive?

_____

_____

3. Do you feel that life is worth living?

_____

_____

4. How satisfied are you with what you have achieved in life?

_____

_____

5. What makes you laugh/cry?

_____

_____

6. What do you fear most? What frightens or upsets you?

_____

_____

7. What goals do you have for the future?

   _____

   _____

8. Do you wish to make any general comments about your attitude toward life?

   _____

   _____

F. Your attitude toward illness, dying, and death

1. What will be important to you when you are dying (e.g., physical comfort, no pain, family members present, etc.)?

   _____

   _____

2. Where do you prefer to die?

   _____

   _____

3. What is your attitude toward death?

   _____

   _____

4. How do you feel about the use of life-sustaining measures in the face of terminal illness?
   Permanent coma _____

   Irreversible chronic illness (e.g., Alzheimer's disease) __

   _____

5. Do you wish to make any general comments about your attitude toward illness, dying, and death?

   _____

   _____

G. Your religious background and beliefs

1. What is your religious background?

   _____

   _____

2. How do your religious beliefs affect your attitude toward serious or terminal illness?

_____

_____

3. Does your attitude toward death find support in your religion?

_____

_____

4. How does your faith community, church, or synagogue view the role of prayer or religious sacraments in an illness?

_____

_____

5. Do you wish to make any general comments about your religious background and beliefs?

_____

_____

H. Your living environment

1. What has been your living situation over the last ten years (e.g., lived alone, lived with others, etc.)?

_____

_____

2. How difficult is it for you to maintain the kind of environment for yourself that you find comfortable? Does any illness or medical problem you have now mean that it will be harder in the future?

_____

_____

3. Do you wish to make any general comments about your living environment?

_____

_____

I. Your attitude toward finances

1. How much do you worry about having enough money to provide for your care?

   _____

   _____

2. Would you prefer to spend less money on your care so that more money can be saved to the benefit of your relatives and/or friends?

   _____

   _____

3. Do you wish to make any general comments about your finances and the cost of health care?

   _____

   _____

J. Your wishes concerning your funeral

1. What are your wishes concerning your funeral and burial or cremation?

   _____

   _____

   _____

2. Have you made funeral arrangements? If so, with whom?

   _____

   _____

   _____

3. Do you have any general comments about how you would like your funeral and burial or cremation to be arranged or conducted?

   _____

   _____

   _____

OPTIONAL QUESTIONS

1. How would you like your obituary (announcement of your death) to read?

   _____

   _____

   _____

   _____

   _____

2. Write yourself a brief eulogy (a statement about yourself to be read at your funeral)

   _____

   _____

   _____

   _____

   _____

Suggestions for Use

After you have completed this form, you may wish to provide copies to your doctors and other health caregivers, your family, your friends, and your attorney. If you have a living will or durable power of attorney for health care decisions, you may wish to attach copies of this form to these documents.

There are other issues to be addressed before a parent dies. You need a crisis plan for what you will do after their death.

The following checklist was developed by Harris McIlwain and his colleagues as part of a 50+ Wellness Plan. It should serve as a basis of discussion. After going through all the issues, you should write the plan down and put it away in a safe place.

CHECKLIST FOR WHEN A PARENT DIES

1. Find instructions for the funeral and burial or cremation. Know whether organs were to be donated for science.

2. Order a dozen certified copies of the death certificate from the county clerk's office or from the funeral director. You will need these to claim death benefits and Social Security as well as to retitle assets and properties if one parent is still alive.

3. File the will in probate court after your lawyer has reviewed it.

4. Apply for death benefits. Call your insurance agent and local Social Security office. If one parent is still alive, you will need a copy of the marriage certificate and both birth certificates.

5. Identify and appropriately dispose of family heirlooms. Hopefully their assignment has been clarified; if not, get help in negotiating such distribution.

6. As money begins to come in from insurance policies and other benefits, deposit this income in short-term bank certificates of deposit. This is not a time to think about investments, and the money will earn some interest for a while.

7. Satisfy debts and notify creditors. Be sure to verify any debt notices as you receive them.

8. Make certain all estate taxes are paid. You must file federal estate taxes within nine months of the death if the estate is larger than $600,000. You must also pay the estate's income tax due by April 15 for every year the estate is open.

9. If one parent is still alive, change all beneficiary designations in the will, insurance policies, investments, retirement plan, and others that named the dead parent as a beneficiary. Have names changed on any joint accounts.

There are many sources of potential financial assistance for burial expenses. Check into the following sources before parents die to see if they qualify:

U.S. Social Security/Canada Pension Benefit

Veterans Administration

Department of Veterans Affairs (Canada)

Union or Employer Pension Fund

Insurance

Workman's Compensation

Fraternal Order of Professional Groups

7. Move on.

Caregivers often report that after their parents have died, they worry about all the things that should have been done for them. Thoughts and feelings about the past well up inside and will not go away. There are three techniques that may be helpful: Practice your worry. Remember the good times. Keep a journal.

Practice your worry. Part of the recovery process for caregivers is to let yourself decompress. Well-intentioned friends and family members may tell you to stop worrying, but that is easier said than done. Remember the techniques discussed in Chapter 3: Allow yourself to worry. Accept the anxiety. Watch the worries. The Japanese Zen master Shunryu Rosh told his students how to calm the mind with the following prescription: "Giving your sheep or cow a large spacious meadow is the way to control him." Give yourself the space for all your worries to roam rather than fight to contain them.

There are several strategies you can use to do this. Set up a time limit to worry. When you feel anxious, take five minutes to do the following:

Sit down and make a list of all your worries. Then speak them all out loud. Keep this up for five minutes, and then stop. Do not contain them. Go back to what you were doing, or get started with another activity.

If possible, find someone you trust to listen to your worries for these five-minute sessions. As you go over your list of worries and exaggerate them with your friend, you may find that your upset gives way to—believe it or not—laughter. The cathartic act of venting your worries combined with the relief of laughter can have what some caregivers describe as a cleansing feeling.

Remember the good times. The second strategy in moving on is to think about your good memories. You can replace your feelings of anxiety and worry about the present with the good feelings associated with a happy memory. The technique is simple. When you feel consumed by your worries, take a five-minute break, but this time close your eyes and think about a time when you felt happiness, triumph, joy, or tenderness. It does not have to be a memory of good times with your parents. When you have locked in on a memory of a time or place, take the next step: Create as many details in your mind as you can, as if you were writing a set of instructions for a movie set or play. Then at the end of five minutes, stop!

Practicing this mind exercise will give you a sense of control about your thoughts. Creating a feeling that you can control the negative and positive thoughts will serve you well through your period of adapting to the end of the caregiving role.

Keep a journal. If you did not keep a diary or journal during the time you were caring for your parents, you can still write one to review what happened. This type of reminiscence can be cathartic because it allows you to relive and review the good times and the bad.

Some caregivers report that this is initially a very painful experience. Sitting down to write can fill you with anxiety or even terror and a desire to run away. Denial is not a one-time experience in caregiving. It is a way of thinking and coping with pain, and the feelings associated with your first entries may be discomforting as you deal with your grief.

Do not force the journal. You may not be ready for it after all. If you cannot get started after a week, put the idea away for a month, but then try it again. This time you may be ready. Some caregivers say it is not so much their painful memories that keep them from writing as that they cannot think of what to write. A helpful way to stimulate your memories is to look through photograph albums or scrapbooks, or to go through your mementos. Looking at these may trigger or stimulate a flood of memories, including details you thought you had forgotten.

Get started on a journal, even if you have never felt that you were particularly good at writing. Buy yourself a notebook and special pen, and choose a period in the day to sit and write for 15 to 30 minutes—more if you have time. It may sound silly to buy a special pen, but this is part of a process of taking control and dedicating yourself to the task.

If you do not have albums or other mementos available, try the following techniques to jar your memories. Make a list of all the things you remember about your childhood home, your grandparents' home, or any other place you can use to anchor yourself somewhere. Then think about happy and pleasant things that you did there, as well as the people who were special to you.

There are also many books to help you, and these can be found in the Selected Readings at the back of this book.

RESOLVING TOUGH FEELINGS

It is not easy for everybody to overcome many of the memories and feelings of caregiving. The most common difficulties for caregivers after their parents die are guilt, prolonged grief, and anger.

Ask yourself the following questions:

- When you think about your parents does your pain, guilt, anger, or anxiety disrupt your work or productivity?

- Do you have sleep problems?

- Do you find yourself ruminating about things you should have handled differently? Do these thoughts occupy your mind more than you think they should?

- Do you find yourself not wanting to face people and activities in your life?

- Do you think you are drinking or eating too much?

- Do you work yourself to exhaustion to keep from thinking about upsetting thoughts?

You may answer yes to most or all of these questions and say to yourself, "So what? It was tough caring for my parents, and it still hurts. It will just take time."

Time *is* the key factor. There is a recovery process after parents have died. Many thoughts and emotions need to be processed. You need time to grieve over your losses, and people grieve in different ways. Some people are very private, while others are more open. Some people think a great deal about what happened, whereas others deal with past events only occasionally. Whatever your style, you need to feel and think about what the loss of your parents means to you. Some people can have such conversations with themselves, but most people need a friend to listen.

Guilt

Caregivers often continue to feel guilt about what they did or did not do for their late parents: They could have brought their mother home instead of placing her in a nursing home. They could have done more when their dad was in the hospital. Such beliefs have the marginal value of allowing people to avoid the feelings of intense helplessness that most people fear more than guilt. Feelings of guilt actually give us the illusion that we have some control of the situation. Guilt is the alternative to the anxiety of feeling totally out of control.

Childhood experiences with parents often set the stage for later feelings of guilt and conscience. Parents in many cultures control children by inducing guilt. Some of us even feel guilty because we took advantage of our parents and got away with a lot in childhood.

Some people feel more guilt than others. It is natural to think about what you did for your parents and to question your behavior, but excessive guilt often appears as self-blame. If you carry a burden of excess guilt, this process of reexamination can become quite destructive. One goal is to forgive yourself. If you think that what you have done is unforgivable, talk about it with friends, family, or others who have also been caregivers. If someone else can understand and forgive you, why not learn to do the same for yourself?

Prolonged Grief and Anger

Mourning for dead parents is both a private and a shared experience. Part of what makes mourning so painful is that you feel that you are alone now. Yet sharing the experience with others is the way you can work through your loss. Mourning is sometimes prolonged, most commonly when people have endured a number of other losses, making them all the more vulnerable.

There are several ways to cope with grief. The most important is not only to talk with people you love and care for about your grief but also to talk about your losses earlier in life. Give yourself permission to grieve. Accept that it will hurt for a while and that you will be depressed, but that this is appropriate. Find a way to deal with your grief with other family members and friends. Make plans for a memorial service or party in your parents' honor. Finding and performing a ritual like a candle-lighting or a daily memorial prayer to celebrate your parents is a very effective way to comfort yourself with the support of those who love you. Rituals will not resolve all of your emotions and grief. They are, however, an important experience in the process of recovery and in working your way into the future a little more knowledgeable about the past and the present.

Selected Readings

This section contains a list of selected books in different areas of interest. Although there are many excellent books on parent-caring, aging, health, and related areas, the ones listed here are those most useful for family caregivers.

Following the reading list are four appendices. Appendix A is a description of programs and services that may be available in your community to help you with the economic, health, social, and welfare needs of your parents. Appendix B provides the addresses and telephone numbers for every state office on aging.

Appendix C lists the addresses and phone numbers of many national, state, and local organizations to help you with information on a wide variety of aging, health, and mental health issues. These organizations are listed here because they have a track record of being responsive to consumers and because of the high quality of written materials available. Many national organizations also have state and local chapters, associations, or societies, and the addresses and phone numbers for these branches are given for the American Psychiatric Association, the American Psychological Association, the National Association of Social Workers, and the National Mental Health Association.

Appendix D lists selected national headquarters or associations concerned with a number of specific diseases or conditions, caregiver/family needs, legal assistance, and long-term care services. We acknowledge the Family Survival Project in San Francisco for compiling most of this list.

Aging: General

Cherlin, Andrew J., and Frank F. Furstenberg. *New American Grandparent: A Place in the Family or Life Apart.* New York: Basic Books, 1986.

Goldman, Connie, and Philip Berman. *The Ageless Spirit.* New York: Ballantine, 1992.

Henig, Robin Marantz, and the editors of *Esquire. How a Woman Ages.* New York: Ballantine, 1985.

Pesmen, Curtis, and the editors of *Esquire. How a Man Ages.* New York: Ballantine, 1984.

Poress, Paula Brown, Diana Laskin Siegel, and the Midlife and Older Women Project. *Ourselves Growing Older.* New York: Touchstone, 1989.

Aging: Inspirational

Beckett, Samuel. *Stirrings Still.* New York: North Star Line, 1991.

Broyard, Anatole. *Intoxicated by My Illness.* New York: Clarkson Potter, 1992.

Fowler, Margaret, and Priscilla McCutcheon. *Songs of Experience: An Anthology of Literature on Growing Old.* New York: Ballantine, 1991.

Hassler, Jon. *Simon's Night. A Novel.* New York: Ballantine, 1979.

Hepburn, Katharine. *Me: Stories of My Life.* New York: Alfred A. Knopf, 1991.

Heynen, Jim, with photographs by Paul Boyer. *One Hundred Over 100.* Golden, Co.: Fulcrum, 1990.

Sarton, May. *Endgame: A Journal of the Seventy-Ninth Year.* New York: W. W. Norton, 1992.

Sennett, Dorothy, ed. *Full Measure: Modern Short Stories on Aging.* St. Paul, Minn.: Graywolf Press, 1988.

Smith, Anita. *The Best of Times.* Birmingham, Ala.: The Best of Times Press, 1989.

Wharton, William. *Dad.* New York: Avon Books, 1981.
York, Pat. *Going Strong.* New York: Arcadia, 1991.

Aging Parents and Children: Inspirational

Anthony, Carolyn, ed. *Family Portraits. Remembrances by Twenty Distinguished Writers.* New York: Penguin, 1989.

Bateson, Mary Catherine. *Composing a Life.* New York: Plume, 1992.

Epstein, H. *Children of the Holocaust: Conversations with Sons and Daughters of Survivors.* New York: G. P. Putnam's Sons, 1979.

Keyes, Ralph. *Sons on Fathers: A Book of Men's Writings.* New York: HarperCollins, 1992.

Malcolm, Andrew. *Someday: The Story of a Mother and Her Son.* New York: Alfred A. Knopf, 1991.

Roth, Philip. *Patrimony.* New York: Simon & Schuster, 1991.

Schreiber, LeAnne. *Midstream: The Story of a Mother's Death and a Daughter's Renewal.* New York: Viking, 1990.

Spiegelman, Art. *Maus I. A Survivor's Tale, My Father Bleeds History?* New York: Pantheon, 1986.

Spiegelman, Art. *Maus II. A Survivor's Tale and How My Troubles Began.* New York: Pantheon, 1992.

Wiesel, Elie. *The Forgotten. A Novel.* New York: Alfred A. Knopf, 1992.

Working with Aging Parents

Akeret, Robert U., with Daniel Klein. *Family Tales, Family Wisdom: How to Gather the Stories of a Life Time and Share Them with Your Family.* New York: William Morrow, 1991.

Edinberg, Mark A. *Talking with Your Aging Parents.* Boston: Shambhala, 1987.

Halpern, James. *Helping Your Aging Parents: A Practical Guide for Adult Children.* New York: McGraw-Hill, 1987.

Jarvik, Lissy F., and Gary Small. *Parent Care.* New York: Bantam, 1990.

Kievman, Beverly, with Susie Blackman. *For Better or For Worse: A Couple's Guide to Dealing with Chronic Illness.* Chicago: Contemporary Books, 1989.

Klagsbrun, Francine. *Mixed Feelings: Love, Hate, Rivalry, and Reconciliation Among Brothers and Sisters.* New York: Bantam, 1992.

Levy, Michael T. *Parenting Mom and Dad.* New York: Prentice-Hall, 1991.

Lustbader, Wendy. *Counting on Kindness.* New York: The Free Press, 1991.

McLean, Helene. *Caring for Your Parents: A Sourcebook of Options and Solutions for Both Generations.* New York, Doubleday, 1987.

Myers, Jane E. *Adult Children and Aging Parents.* Dubuque, Ia.: Kendall/Hunt, 1989.

Rob, Caroline. *The Caregiver's Guide.* Boston: Houghton Mifflin, 1991.

Shelley, Florence. *When Your Parents Grow Old.* 2nd ed. New York: Harper & Row, 1988.

Silverstone, Barbara, and Helen Kendel Hyman. *You and Your Aging Parent: A Family Guide to Emotional, Physical, and Financial Problems.* 3rd ed. New York: Pantheon, 1989.

When Caregiving Is Traumatic

Caterall, Don R. *Back From the Brink: A Family Guide to Overcoming Traumatic Stress.* New York: Quantum, 1992.

Colgrove, M., H. Bloonfield, and P. McWilliams. *How to Survive the Loss of a Love.* New York: Bantam, 1976.

Hewett, J. H. *After Suicide.* Louisville, Ky.: Westminster John Knox, 1980.

When Parents Have Hurt You

Bass, E., and L. Davis. *The Courage to Heal.* New York: Harper & Row, 1988.

Gil, E. *Outgrowing the Pain: A Book For and About Adults Abused as Children.* San Francisco: Launch Press, 1983.

Whitfield, C. L. *Healing the Child Within: Discovery and Recovery for Adult Children of Dysfunctional Families.* Deerfield Beach, Fla.: Health Communications, 1987.

Mastering Emotions

Beck, Aaron T., and Gary Emery, with Ruth C. Greenberg. *Anxiety Disorders and Phobias*. New York: Basic Books, 1983.

Davis, M., E. R. Eshelmon, and M. McKay. *The Relaxation and Stress Reduction Workbook*. Oakland, Calif.: New Harbinger, 1985.

Hall, Lindsey, and Leigh Cohn. *Self Esteem: Tools for Recovery*. Carlsbad, Calif.: Gurze, 1990.

Johnson, V. *I'll Quit Tomorrow*. New York: Harper & Row, 1980.

Klein, Donald, and Paul Wender. *Understanding Depression*. New York: Oxford, 1993.

Lerner, H. G. *The Dance of Anger*. New York: Harper & Row, 1985.

Manttsky, M. C. *Coping Better . . . Anytime, Anywhere*. New York: Simon & Schuster, 1986.

Manttsky, M. C., and A. Hendricks. *You and Your Emotions*. Lexington, Ky.: Rational Self-Help Aids. (Write I'ACT, 3939 West Spencer Street, Appleton, WI 54914.)

McKay, Matthew. *When Anger Hurts*. Oakland, Calif.: New Harbinger, 1989.

McKay, Matthew, and Patrick Fanning. *Self-Esteem*. Oakland, Calif.: New Harbinger, 1990.

Neeld, Elizabeth Harper. *Seven Choices: Taking the Steps to New Life After Losing Someone You Love*. New York: Potter, 1992.

Ryan, Regina Sara. *The Fine Art of Recuperation: A Guide to Surviving and Thriving After Illness, Accident, or Surgery*. Los Angeles: Jeremy P. Tarcher, 1989.

Seligman, Martin. *Learned Optimism*. New York: Alfred A. Knopf, 1991.

Tavris, Carol. *Anger*. New York: Touchstone, 1986.

Conflict Resolution

Adizes, Ichak. *Mastering Change*. Santa Monica, Calif.: Adizes Institute, 1992.

Tannen, Deborah. *You Just Don't Understand: Women and Men in Conversation*. New York: Ballantine, 1990.

Weeks, Dudley. *Eight Essential Steps to Conflict Resolution.* Los Angeles: Jeremy P. Tarcher, 1991.

Taking Care of Yourself: Exercise and Diet

Finn, Susan, and Linda Stern Kass. *The Real Life Nutrition Book.* New York: Penguin, 1992.

McIlwain, Harris H., Cori F. Steinmeyer, Debra Fulghum Bruce, R. E. Fulghum, and Robert G. Bruce. *The 50+ Wellness Plan: A Complete Program for Maintaining Nutritional, Financial and Emotional Well-Being for Mature Adults.* New York: John Wiley & Sons, 1990.

Stare, Frederick, and Virginia Aronson. *Food for Fitness After Fifty: A Menu For Good Health in Later Years.* Philadelphia: George F. Stickley, 1985.

Medical Conditions

Abrams, William B., and Robert Berkow, eds. *The Merck Manual of Geriatrics.* Rahway, N.J.: Merck, Sharp & Dohme Research Laboratories, 1990.

Aspen Reference Group. *Geriatric Patient Education Resource Manual.* Frederick, Md.: Aspen, 1982.

Beers, Mark H., and Stephen K. Urice. *Aging in Good Health: A Complete Essential Medical Guide for Older Men and Women and Their Families.* New York: Pocket Books, 1992.

Roe, Daphne. *Geriatric Nutrition.* 3rd ed. Englewood Cliffs, N.J.: Prentice-Hall, 1992.

Solomon, David H., Elyse Salend, Anna Nolan Rahman, Marie Bolduc Liston, and David B. Reuben. *A Consumer's Guide to Aging.* Baltimore: The Johns Hopkins University Press, 1992.

Housing

Carlin, Vivian F., and Ruth Mansberg. *Where Can Mom Live? A Family Guide to Living Arrangements for Elderly Patients.* Lexington, Mass.: Lexington Books, 1987.

Consumer Reports. *Communities for the Elderly* (February 1990), pp. 123–31.

Golant, Stephen M. *Housing America's Elderly: Many Possibilities/ Few Choices.* Newbury Park, Calif.: Sage Publications, 1992.

Mathews, Joseph. *Elder Care: A Consumer's Guide to Choosing and Financing Long Term Care.* Berkeley, Calif.: Nolo Press, 1991.

Finances

Mathews, Joseph. *Social Security, Medicine, and Pensions.* Berkeley, Calif.: Nolo Press, 1992.

Smith, Wesley J. *The Senior Citizens Handbook.* Los Angeles: Price Stern Sloan, 1989.

Weltman, Barbara. *Your Parent's Financial Search.* New York: John Wiley & Sons, 1992.

Home Care and Adult Day Care

Crichton, Jen. *Age Care Sourcebook: A Resource Guide for the Aging and Their Families.* New York: Simon & Schuster, 1987.

Golden, Susan. *Nursing a Loved One at Home: A Caregiver's Guide.* Philadelphia: Running Press, 1988.

Nassif, Janet Zhun. *Home Health Care Solution: A Complete Consumer Guide.* New York: Harper & Row, 1985.

On Lok Senior Health Services. *Directory of Adult Day Care in America.* Washington, D.C.: Nutritional Council on Aging, 1987.

Nursing Homes

Goldsmith, Seth B. *Choosing a Nursing Home.* New York: Prentice-Hall, 1990.

Hughes, Marylou. *The Nursing Home Experience: A Family Guide to Making It Better.* New York: Continuum, 1992.

Meskinsky, Joanne. *How to Choose a Nursing Home: A Guide to Quality Caring.* New York: Avon, 1991.

Mongean, S., ed. *Directory of Nursing Homes.* 3rd ed. Phoenix, Ariz.: Oryx Press, 1988.

Peck, M. Scott. *A Bed by the Window.* New York: Bantam, 1991.

Richards, Marty. *Choosing a Nursing Home: A Guidebook for Families.* Seattle: University of Washington Press, 1985.

Decisions About Medical Care and Dying

Dubler, Nancy, and David Nimmons. *Ethics on Call: A Medical Ethicist Shows How to Take Charge of Life-and-Death Choices.* New York: Harmony Books, 1982.

Flynn, Eileen P. *Your Living Will: Why, When and How to Write One.* New York: Citadel Press, 1992.

Kastenbaum, Robert. *The Psychology of Death.* New York: Springer, 1992.

Sankar, Andrea. *Dying at Home.* Baltimore: The Johns Hopkins University Press, 1991.

Alzheimer's Disease and Related Disorders

Cohen, Donna, and Carl Eisdorfer. *The Loss of Self: A Family Resource for Alzheimer's Disease.* New York: W. W. Norton, 1986.

Coughlan, Patricia Brown. *Facing Alzheimer's: Family Caregivers Speak.* New York: Ballantine, 1993.

Gruetzner, Howard. *Alzheimer's: A Caregiver's Guide and Sourcebook.* New York: John Wiley & Sons, 1992.

Mace, Nancy, and Peter Rabins. *The 36-Hour Day.* Baltimore: The Johns Hopkins University Press, 1981.

Children's Books: Aging and Aging Families

Brodsky, Beverly. *The Story of Job.* New York: George Braziller, 1986.

Capote, Truman. *I Remember Grandpa.* Atlanta: Peachtree Publications, 1985.

Gellman, Marc, and Thomas Hartman. *Where Does God Live? Questions and Answers for Parents and Children.* New York: Triumph Books, 1991.

Borltzer, Etan. *What Is God?* Toronto: Firefly Books, 1989.

Legal Issues

American Bar Association. *Personal and Estate Planning for the Elderly.* Chicago: ABA, 1989.

American Bar Association, Commission on Legal Problems of the Elderly. *Law and Aging Resource Guide.* Washington, D.C.: ABA, 1987.

Regan, J. J. *Your Legal Rights in Later Life.* Glenview, Ill.: Scott, Foresman & Co., 1989.

Drugs

Conolly, Matthew, and Michael Orme. *The Patient's Desk Reference: Thousands of Medications Indexed by Illness.*

Gorman, Jack M. *The Essential Guide to Psychiatric Drugs.* New York: St. Martin's Press, 1990.

Roe, Daphne. *Handbook on Drug and Nutrient Interactions.* Chicago: American Dietetic Association, 1989.

Appendix A

PROGRAMS AND SERVICES IN YOUR COMMUNITY

There are a number of social programs and community services that can address your parents' economic, health, social, and welfare needs. This appendix is not intended to be a complete listing of them, but it is a guide to programs and services that exist in a number of communities around the United States. Some, like Social Security or congregate meals, are usually available everywhere, but others, such as transportation or adult day care, may have long waiting lists. Other programs may have complicated application procedures, be restricted to persons who are very poor, or simply not exist in your community.

For information about these programs and services, contact the office of aging in your state listed in Appendix B or the area agency on aging in your community, listed in your telephone book.

SOCIAL SECURITY

Social Security is a retirement income supplement available to most older Americans. To get information, call your local Social Security office listed in your telephone book, or the Social Security Administration office toll-free at 1-800-772-1213.

SUPPLEMENTAL SECURITY INCOME (SSI)

The Supplemental Security Income Program, which is administered by the Social Security Administration, guarantees a minimum amount of cash income to older, blind, and disabled individuals who have very low incomes and few assets. For instructions about eligibility and benefits, contact your local Social Security office.

MEDICARE

Medicare is a federal health insurance program to help with many of the medical expenses of Americans sixty-five and older. Those who are eligible for Social Security may apply for Medicare benefits. Your parents can apply for Medicare benefits three months before their sixty-fifth birthdays.

Medicare has two parts. Part A is hospital insurance, which helps pay the cost of care when you are a hospital inpatient. Part A also helps with limited inpatient care in a skilled nursing facility, home care, and hospice care under certain conditions. But Medicare does not cover many long-term care services. You can get pamphlets with information about Medicare benefits from your local Social Security office. The number of days Medicare pays for hospital care is determined by a system based upon patient diagnosis and the medical indications for hospital care. The discharge process will be started by your parents' physician when it is determined that it is no longer medically necessary for them to stay in the hospital. If your parents or you do not agree with the discharge decision, you can appeal. To start the appeal you must contact the Peer Review Organization (PRO) in your state, which is responsible for reviewing hospital services. You can find out the name, address, and phone number for the PRO in your area from the hospital administration office or business office, or from the social service office in your community. When you call the PRO office, ask how you can start the appeal and whether there is a time limit.

Medicare Part B is medical insurance to help pay for certain doctors' services, hospital outpatient procedures, and a few other medical services. Your parents must enroll in Part B and pay a monthly premium to receive Part B services.

Contact your local Social Security office, listed in the yellow or blue pages of your telephone book, to apply for Medicare or to ask questions about it.

MEDICAID

Medicaid is a program that provides medical assistance to low-income individuals who are aged, blind, and disabled, as well as certain families with children. Medicaid is financed by federal and state matching funds.

Some states provide funds for persons who are deemed medically needy. *Medically needy* persons are defined as those whose income is considered sufficient to cover living expenses but not large enough to pay for medical care. Since the income levels that signify medical neediness are set by each state, people with the same incomes and resources may be eligible for Medicaid in one state but not in another.

In 1981 Congress passed legislation giving the Health Care Financing Administration (HCFA) authority to waive some Medicaid requirements so that states could increase their funding for community services for people who would be institutionalized in a nursing home without such services. The services covered under these Medicaid Home and Community-Based Waivers include case management, home health aid, personal care, adult day care, respite care, rehabilitation, and other services.

For information on Medicaid, contact your local county welfare office, listed in the yellow or blue pages of your telephone book.

CONGREGATE NUTRITION AND HOME-DELIVERED MEAL PROGRAMS

Under the Older Americans Act, passed by Congress in 1965, federal funds are distributed through states to provide meals to older persons sixty years of age and older. Congregate nutrition programs now operate in all fifty states. No person is refused on the basis of ability to contribute, and most of these programs accept food stamps. Most congregate programs are located in senior centers or other community sites such as churches, schools, or community centers. Besides providing meals, many of these nutrition sites offer services such as nutrition education, special diets, shopping assistance, food co-ops, and mobile food markets.

Home-delivered meal programs, also authorized by the Older Americans Act, provide meals to persons sixty and older who are homebound. These programs are commonly known as Meals on Wheels. Some home-delivered programs also provide liquid nutrition supplements or other food items.

NATIVE AMERICAN SERVICES

The Older Americans Act specifically established services to meet the special needs of older American Indians on Indian reservations as well as older Hawaiian natives. Funds are available to Indian tribes and native

Hawaiian organizations who represent at least fifty Indian or native Hawaiians sixty years and older.

Adult Day Care

There are two forms of adult day care—adult day health care and adult day social care. Adult day health care provides services to frail and/or disabled adults in a group setting to prevent institutionalization. Services offered include health monitoring, rehabilitation, occupational therapy, personal care, transportation, and a noon meal. Adult day health care can be publicly or privately sponsored, and many Medicaid-eligible older persons can access this program.

Social day care, usually at senior centers, provides frail older persons with social or recreational care in organized group programs. It usually includes transportation and a noon meal.

Senior Centers

There are more than 12,000 senior centers across the United States, and all of them offer social and recreational programs. Many senior centers serve as community centers for many services, including meals, adult education classes, day care, health screening, transportation, social services, and many other programs. These centers usually offer other services at little or no cost.

Transportation Services

Transportation is one of the most important yet often unavailable services. Taking a relative from one location to another should be simple and affordable, but it is not. In some communities public, private, or volunteer groups provide transportation for older persons to make medical appointments or to go shopping.

Case Management Services

Case management services match the available services to an individual's needs. Case management services for long-term care usually include the following four components.

- screening and assessment to determine whether an individual needs and is eligible for a specific service;

- development of a care plan with the types and amounts of care to be provided;

- reassessment of the continuing need for services.

Case management services are provided by many different community organizations such as home health agencies, area agencies on aging, and other social and health agencies in the community. Some states, such as Illinois and Oregon, have statewide long-term care systems where one agency in the community performs case management services.

In-Home Health Aid/Personal Care Services

These services are usually medical or personal care services provided by a trained person under the supervision of a licensed medical professional such as a registered nurse (RN), licensed practical nurse (LPN), or therapist.

Eligibility is usually the same as qualifications for Medicaid services includes:

- hair care, dentures, personal hygiene

- activities of daily living—bathing, dressing, grooming, eating, toileting

- taking medications

- exercise

- skin care

- changing dressings

- trips to a physician's office for medical diagnoses or treatment

- assistance with shopping

- assistance with meal preparation

- supervision for clients who cannot be left alone.

Homemaker/Chore Services

These nonmedical services help older persons with many tasks associated with keeping a home or household. Examples of these services include:

- escorting or transport of clients to medical care services

- shopping for food, clothes, and other needs
- running important errands
- washing, drying, ironing, mending clothes, or helping clients to do same
- housework
- preparing meals
- assisting with eating.

A number of other services help clients bathe, dress, toilet, and get around. Such services are available at no cost for those who meet eligibility requirements, and in some communities they may be available to others using a sliding scale for payment.

Minor Home Repair Services

Many communities offer minor home repair services for older persons so they may continue to live at home in safety and comfort. These services include:

- repairing faucets, pipes, drains, and toilets
- replacing switches, wall sockets, and fixtures
- rebuilding broken windows
- replacing broken windows
- building wheelchair ramps
- installing doors, locks, grab bars, and handrails.

Volunteer Programs

ACTION is a federal volunteer organization that administers three volunteer programs for older persons: the Senior Companions Program, the Foster Grandparent Program, and the Retired Senior Volunteer Program.

The Retired Senior Volunteer Program and the Foster Grandparent Program provide small nontaxable stipends, meals, and transportation cost reimbursement, and insurance for part-time jobs. Volunteers in the Senior Companions work only with homebound and frail older persons, whereas the Foster Grandparents work with children who have special needs. To be eligible for either of these programs, your parents must be at least sixty years old and have an income less than 125 percent of the poverty level.

The Retired Senior Volunteer Program (RSVP) is the largest of the ACTION volunteer programs. Although there is no stipend, meals, transportation, and insurance are provided. RSVP volunteers work twenty hours a week in community settings such as senior centers, nutrition programs, schools, and other sites.

Appendix B

STATE AGENCIES ON AGING

Alabama
Commission on Aging. 770 Washington Avenue, Suite 470, Montgomery AL 36130. (205) 242-5743

Alaska
Older Alaskans Commission. 333 Willoughby Avenue, Department of Administration, P.O. Box 110209, Juneau AK 99811-0209. (907) 465-3250

Arizona
Aging and Adult Administration, Department of Economic Security. 1789 West Jefferson, 2SW, 950A, Phoenix AZ 85007. (602) 542-4446

Arkansas
Division of Aging and Adult Services, Arkansas Department of Human Services. 7th and Main Street, P.O. Box 1437, Slot 1412, Little Rock AR 72201. (501) 682-2441

California
Department of Aging, Health and Welfare Agency. 1600 K Street, Sacramento CA 95814. (916) 322-5290

Colorado
Aging and Adult Services, Department of Social Services. 1575 Sherman Street, Denver CO 80203-1714. (303) 866-3851

Connecticut
Department on Aging. 175 Main Street, Hartford CT 06106. (203) 566-3238

Delaware
Division on Aging, Department of Health and Social Services. 1901 North Dupont Highway, New Castle DE 19720. (302) 577-4971

District of Columbia
District of Columbia Office on Aging. 1424 K Street N.W., Second Floor, Washington DC 20005. (202) 724-5622

Florida
Program Office of Aging and Adult Services, Department of Elder Affairs. Building 1, Room 317, 1317 Winewood Boulevard, Tallahassee FL 32399-0700. (904) 922-5297

Georgia
Office of Aging, Department of Human Resources. 878 Peachtree Street N.E., Room 632, Atlanta GA 30309. (404) 894-5333

Hawaii
Executive Office on Aging, Office of the Governor, State of Hawaii. 335 Merchant Street, Room 241, Honolulu HI 96813. (808) 586-0100

Idaho
Idaho Office on Aging. Statehouse—Room 108, Boise ID 83720. (208) 334-3833

Illinois
Department on Aging. 421 East Capitol Avenue, Springfield IL 62701. (217) 785-2870

Indiana
Aging/In-Home Services, Department on Aging and Rehabilitative Services. 402 West Washington Street, Room W454, P.O. Box 7083, Indianapolis IN 46204. (317) 232-7020

Iowa
Commission on Aging. Jewett Building, Suite 236, 914 Grand Avenue, Des Moines IA 50319. (515) 281-5187

Kansas
Department on Aging. Docking State Office Building, 122 S., 915 S.W. Harrison, Topeka KS 66612. (913) 296-4986

Kentucky
Division for Aging Services, Bureau of Social Services. 275 East Main Street, Frankfort KY 40601. (502) 564-6930

Louisiana
Office of Elderly Affairs. P.O. Box 80374, 4550 North Boulevard, 2nd Floor, Baton Rouge LA 70806. (504) 925-1700

Maine
Bureau of Elder and Adult Services, Department of Human Services. State House, Station 11, 35 Anthony Avenue, Augusta ME 04333. (207) 626-5335

Maryland
Office on Aging. State Office Building, 301 West Preston Street, Room 1004, Baltimore MD 21201. (410) 225-1100

Massachusetts
Executive Office of Elder Affairs. One Ashburton Place, 5th Floor, Boston MA 02108. (617) 727-7750

Michigan
Office of Services for the Aging. P.O. Box 30026, Lansing MI 48909. (517) 373-8230

Minnesota
Board on Aging. 444 Lafayette Road, St. Paul MN 55155-3843. (612) 296-2770

Mississippi
Council on Aging, Division of Aging and Adult Services. 455 North Lamar Street, Jackson MS 39202. (601) 359-6770

Missouri
Division of Aging, Department of Social Services. 615 Howerton Court, P.O. Box 1337, Jefferson City MO 65109. (314) 751-3082

Montana
The Governor's Office on Aging. State Capitol Building, Capitol Station, Room 219, Helena MT 59620. (406) 444-3111

Nebraska
Department on Aging. P.O. Box 95044, 301 Centennial Mall South, Lincoln NE 68509. (402) 471-2306

Nevada
Aging Services/Human Resources. 340 North 11 Street, Suite 114, Las Vegas NV 89101. (702) 486-3545

New Hampshire
Division of Elderly and Adult Services. 6 Hazen Drive, Concord NH 03301. (603) 271-4394

New Jersey
Division on Aging, Department of Community Affairs. CN 807, South Broad and Front Street, Trenton NJ 08625-0807. (609) 292-4833

New Mexico
State Agency on Aging. LaVilla Rivera Building, 224 East Palace Avenue, Santa Fe NM 87501. (505) 827-7640

New York
Office for the Aging. New York State Plaza, Agency Building 2, Albany NY 12223. (518) 474-4425

North Carolina
Division on Aging. 693 Palmer Drive, Raleigh NC 27626-0531. (919) 733-3983

North Dakota
Aging Services Division, Department of Human Services. 1929 North Washington Street, P.O. Box 7070, Bismarck ND 58507-7070. (701) 224-2577 or (800) 472-2622

Ohio
Ohio Department on Aging. 50 West Broad Street, 8th Floor, Columbus OH 43266-0501. (614) 466-5500

Oklahoma
Aging Services Division, Department of Human Services. P.O. Box 25352, Oklahoma City OK 73125. (405) 521-2281

Oregon
Senior & Disabled Services Division. 500 Summer Street, N.E., 2nd Floor North, Salem OR 97310-1015. (503) 378-4728

Pennsylvania
Department of Aging. Market Street State Office Building, 7th Floor, 400 Market Street, Harrisburg PA 17101-2301. (717) 783-1550

Rhode Island
Department of Elderly Affairs. 160 Pine Street, Providence RI 02903-3708. (401) 277-2858

South Carolina
Commission on Aging. 400 Arbor Lake Drive, Suite B-500, Columbia SC 29223. (803) 735-0210

South Dakota
Office of Adult Services and Aging. 700 Governors Drive, Pierre SD 57501. (605) 773-3656

Tennessee
Commission on Aging. 706 Church Street, Suite 201, Nashville TN 37243-0860. (615) 741-2056

Texas
Department on Aging. 1949 IH-35 South, P.O. Box 12786, Austin TX 78711-3702. (512) 444-2727

Utah
Division of Aging and Adult Services, Department of Human Services. 2001 South State Street, Room S-1500, Salt Lake City UT 84190-2300. (801) 468-2454

Vermont
Department of Aging and Disabilities. 103 South Main Street, Waterbury VT 05671-2301. (802) 241-2400

Virginia
Department for the Aging. 700 East Franklin Street, 10th Floor, Richmond VA 23219-2327. (804) 225-2271

Washington
Aging and Adult Services Administration, Social and Health Services. P.O. Box 45600, Olympia WA 98504-5600. (206) 493-2500

West Virginia
Commission on Aging. Holly Grove, 1900 Kanawha Boulevard, East, Charleston WV 25305-0160. (304) 558-3317

Wisconsin
Bureau on Aging, Division of Community Services. P.O. Box 7851, Madison WI 53707. (608) 266-2536

Wyoming
Commission on Aging. Hathaway Building, Room 139, Cheyenne WY 82002. (307) 777-7986

American Samoa
Territorial Administration on Aging. Office of the Governor, Pago Pago, American Samoa 96799. (684) 633-1252

Guam
Guam Division of Senior Citizens, Department of Public Health and Social Services. P.O. Box 2816, Agana, GU 96910. (671) 632-4141

Puerto Rico
Governor's Office of Elderly Affairs. Cubian Plaza Stop 23, U.M. Floor, Office C, Ponce de Leon Avenue, #1603, Santurce, PR 00908. (809) 721-5710

Virgin Islands
Senior Citizens Affairs, Department of Human Services. #19 Estate Diamond, Frederiksted, St. Croix, VI 00840. (809) 772-4950

Appendix C

NATIONAL, STATE, AND LOCAL ORGANIZATIONS PROVIDING INFORMATION AND SERVICES

These national, state, and local organizations and professional groups concerned with aging, health, and mental health issues are listed here because of their importance, responsiveness to people looking for information, and the usefulness of their written materials.

NATIONAL RESOURCES

Alcoholics Anonymous (AA). General Service Board of Alcoholics Anonymous, P.O. Box 459, Grand Central Station, New York NY 10163. (212) 686-1100

The Alzheimer's Association (formerly The Alzheimer's Disease and Related Disorders Association). 919 N. Michigan Ave., 10th floor, Chicago IL 60611. (800) 272-3900; (312) 335-8700

American Association for Geriatric Psychiatry. P.O. Box 376A, Greenbelt MD 20770. (301) 220-0952

American Association of Retired Persons. 1909 K Street N.W., Washington DC 20049. (202) 728-4300

American Dietetic Association. 216 West Jackson Boulevard, Suite 800, Chicago IL 60606-6995. (800) 366-1655

The American Geriatrics Society. 770 Lexington Avenue, Suite 400, New York NY 10021. (212) 308-1414

American Psychiatric Association. 1400 K Street N. W., Washington DC 20009. (202) 682-6220

American Psychological Association. 1200 17th Street N. W., Washington DC 20036. (202) 955-7600

American Society on Aging. 833 Market Street, Suite 512, San Francisco CA 94103. (415) 543-2617

The Department of Veterans Affairs. 810 Vermont Avenue N. W., Washington DC 20420. (202) 737-5050

Family Service of America. 11700 West Lake Park Drive, Park Place, Milwaukee WI 53224. (414) 359-1040

Gerontological Society of America. 1411 K Street N. W., Suite 300, Washington DC 20005. (202) 393-1411

National Alliance for the Mentally Ill. 2101 Wilson Boulevard, Suite 302, Arlington VA 22201. (703) 524-7600

National Association of Area Agencies on Aging. 600 Maryland Avenue S. W., Washington DC 20024. (202) 484-7520

National Association of Social Workers. 7981 Eastern Avenue, Silver Spring MD 29010. (301) 565-0333

National Council of Community Mental Health Centers. 12300 Twinbrook Parkway, Suite 320, Rockville MD 20852. (301) 984-6200

National Depressive and Manic Depressive Association. Merchandise Mart, Box 3395, Chicago IL 60654. (312) 939-2442

The National Institute of Mental Health. 5600 Fishers Lane, Rockville MD 20857. (301) 443-3367

National Institute on Aging, National Institutes of Health. Bethesda MD 20892. (301) 496-9322

National Institute on Aging Information Center. P.O. Box 8057, Gaithersburg MD 20898-8057. (301) 495-3455

National Mental Health Association. 1021 Prince Street, Alexandria VA 22314-2971. (703) 684-7722

National Mental Health Consumers' Self-Help Clearinghouse. 311 South Juniper Street, Suite 902, Philadelphia PA 19107. (215) 735-6367

STATE RESOURCES

American Psychiatric Association: Local Psychiatric Societies

Alabama
Alabama Psychiatric Society. P.O. Box 66311, Birmingham AL 35210. (205) 933-7724

Alaska
Alaska District Branch of the American Psychiatric Association. 4001 Dale Street, No. 101, Anchorage AK 99508. (907) 561-1361

Arizona
Arizona Psychiatric Society. Desert Vista Hospital, 570 West Brown Road, Mesa AZ 85201. (602) 898-3314

Arkansas
Arkansas Psychiatric Society. UAMS Department of Psychiatry, 4301 West Markham, Slot 554, Little Rock AR 72205. (501) 661-5587

California
Central California Psychiatric Society. 748 Plum Lane, Davis CA 95616. (916) 753-2401

Northern California Psychiatric Society. 1631 Ocean Avenue, San Francisco CA 94112. (415) 334-2418

Orange County Psychiatric Society. 300 South Flower Street, P.O. Box 1297, Orange CA 92668. (714) 978-3016

San Diego Society of Psychiatric Physicians. 7159 Navajo Road, No. 120, San Diego CA 92119. (619) 582-3221.

Southern California Psychiatric Society. 2601 Ocean Park Boulevard, Suite 314, Santa Monica CA 90405. (213) 450-4610

Colorado
Colorado Psychiatric Society. 5991 South Bellaire Way, Littleton CO 80121. (303) 220-9565

Connecticut
Connecticut Psychiatric Society. One Regency Drive, P.O. Box 30, Bloomfield CT 06002. (203) 243-3977

Delaware
Delaware Psychiatric Association. Academy of Medicine Building, 1925 Lovering Avenue, Wilmington DE 19806. (302) 428-2961

District of Columbia
Washington Psychiatric Society. 1400 K Street N.W., Washington DC 20005. (202) 682-6192

Florida
Florida Psychiatric Society. P.O. Box 10002, Tallahassee FL 32302. (904) 222-8404

South Florida Psychiatric Society, Inc. P.O. Box 331266, Miami FL 33133. (305) 854-6802

Georgia
Georgia Psychiatric Association. 938 Peachtree Street N.E., Atlanta GA 30309. (404) 876-7535

Hawaii
Hawaii Psychiatric Society. 3879 Lurline Drive, Honolulu HI 96816. (808) 732-3304

Idaho
Idaho District Branch of the American Psychiatric Association. 339 North Allumbaugh, Boise ID 83704. (208) 323-1125

Illinois
Illinois Psychiatric Society. 20 North Michigan Avenue, Suite 700. Chicago IL 60602. (312) 263-7391

Indiana
Indiana Psychiatric Society. 5331 Glen Stewart Way, Indianapolis IN 46254. (317) 293-4770

Northern Indiana Psychiatric Society. 701 Wall Street, Valparaiso IN 46383. (219) 464-8541

Iowa
Iowa Psychiatric Society. 1001 Grand Avenue, West Des Moines IA 50265. (515) 223-1401

Kansas
Kansas Psychiatric Society. 1259 Pembroke Lane, Topeka KS 66604. (913) 232-5985

Kentucky
Kentucky Psychiatric Association. P.O. Box 198, Frankfort KY 40602. (502) 695-4843

Louisiana
Lousiana Psychiatric Association. P.O. Box 15765, New Orleans LA 70175. (504) 891-1030

Maine
Maine Psychiatric Association. RFD No. 1., P.O. Box 1620, North White-field ME 04353. (207) 549-5786

Maryland
Maryland Psychiatric Society, Inc. 1204 Maryland Avenue, Baltimore MD 21201. (301) 625-0232

Massachusetts
Massachusetts Psychiatric Society. One Washington Street, Suite 210, Wellesley MA 02181. (617) 237-8100

Michigan
Michigan Psychiatric Society. 21700 Northwestern Highway, Suite 1150, Southfield MI 48075. (313) 552-8666

Minnesota
Minnesota Psychiatric Society. 1770 Colvin Avenue, St. Paul MN 55116. (612) 698-1971

Mississippi
Mississippi Psychiatric Association. Mississippi State Medical Association, 735 Riverside Drive, P.O. Box 5229, Jackson MS 39216. (601) 354-5433

Missouri
Central Missouri Psychiatric Society. 2401 Bernadette, Suite 204, Columbia MO 65203-4672. (314) 445-6444

Eastern Missouri Psychiatric Society. 3839 Lindell Boulevard, St. Louis MO 63108. (314) 371-5226

Western Missouri District Branch of the American Psychiatric Association. 3036 Gillham Road, Kansas City MO 64108. (816) 531-8432

Montana
Montana Psychiatric Association. College Professional Building, 2520 17th Street West, Billings MT 59102. (406) 259-1425

Nebraska
Nebraska Psychiatric Society. Immanuel Hospital, 6901 North 72nd Street, Omaha NE 68122. (402) 572-2907

Nevada
Nevada Association of Psychiatric Physicians. The Montevista Center, 5900 West Rochelle Avenue, Las Vegas NV 89103. (702) 364-1111 ext. 103

New Hampshire
New Hampshire Psychiatric Society. 76 South State Street, P.O. Box 1382, Concord NH 03302. (603) 228-1231

New Jersey
New Jersey Psychiatric Association. 803 Partridge Drive, Bridgewater NJ 08807. (201) 685-0650

New Mexico
Psychiatric Medical Association of New Mexico. P.O. Box 26666, Albuquerque NM 87125. (505) 841-3511

New York
Bronx District Branch of the American Psychiatric Association. 78 Woodcrest Avenue, White Plains NY 10604. (914) 946-3105

Brooklyn Psychiatric Society, Inc. Four Chimney Court, Brookhaven NY 11719. (516) 286-8907

Central New York District Branch of the American Psychiatric Association. 122 Orvilton Drive, DeWitt NY 13214. (315) 446-0944

Genesee Valley Psychiatric Association. 16 North Goodman Street, Rochester NY 14607. (716) 461-2155

Mid-Hudson District Branch of the American Psychiatric Association. 141 Van Wagner Road, Poughkeepsie NY 12603. (914) 452-5894

Nassau Psychiatric Society. 400 Sunrise Highway, Amityville NY 11701. (516) 691-8080

New York County District Branch of the American Psychiatric Association. 150 East 58th Street, 16th Floor, New York NY 10022. (212) 421-4732/33/34

New York State Capital District Branch of the American Psychiatric Association. P.O. Box 5, New Baltimore NY 12121. (518) 756-8149

Northern New York District Branch of the American Psychiatric Association. 1400 Noyes Street, Utica NY 13502. (315) 797-6800

Queens County District Branch of the American Psychiatric Association. 47-04 159th Street, Flushing NY 11358. (718) 461-8413

Suffolk County District Branch of the American Psychiatric Association. 36 Old Landers Court, Smithtown NY 11787. (516) 265-5134

West Hudson District Branch of the American Psychiatric Association. 36 College Avenue, Nanuet NY 10954. (914) 358-1687

Westchester County District Branch of the American Psychiatric Association. Erie County Medical Center, 78 Woodcrest Avenue, White Plains NY 10604. (914) 946-9008

Western New York Psychiatric Society. 462 Grider Street, Buffalo NY 14215. (716) 898-3251

North Carolina
North Carolina Psychiatric Association. 4917 Waters Edge Drive, Suite 250, Raleigh NC 27606. (919) 859-3370

North Dakota
North Dakota District Branch of the American Psychiatric Association. 700 First Avenue South, Fargo ND 58103. (701) 235-5354

Ohio
Ohio Psychiatric Association. c/o Ohio State Medical Association, 600 South High Street, Columbus OH 43215. (614) 228-6971

Oklahoma
Oklahoma Psychiatric Association. P.O. Box 1328, Norman OK 73070. (405) 321-4514

Oregon
Oregon Psychiatric Association. 1700 S.W. Columbia, Portland OR 97201. (503) 224-6364

Pennsylvania
Pennsylvania Psychiatric Society. 20 Erford Road, Lemoyne PA 17043. (717) 763-7151

Puerto Rico
Puerto Rico Psychiatric Society. Mepsi Center, Call Box 6089, Bayamón PR 00621-6089. (809) 793-3030

Rhode Island
Rhode Island Psychiatric Society. 204 Taber Avenue, Providence RI 02906. (401) 246-1195

South Carolina
South Carolina Psychiatric Association. 1214 Henderson Street, Columbia SC 29201. (803) 765-1498

South Dakota
South Dakota Psychiatric Association. 800 East 21st Street, Sioux Falls SD 57101. (605) 339-6785

Tennessee
Tennessee Psychiatric Association. 112 Louise Avenue, Nashville TN 37203. (615) 478-0605

Texas
Texas Society of Psychiatric Physicians. 400 West 15th Street, Suite 1018, Austin TX 78701. (512) 478-0605

Utah
Utah Psychiatric Association. 540 East 500 South, Salt Lake City UT 84108. (801) 355-7477

Vermont
Vermont Psychiatric Association. c/o Thomas Chittenden Health Center, Williston VT 05495. (802) 879-0242

Virginia
Psychiatric Society of Virginia. 209 Culpepper Road, Richmond VA 23229. (804) 282-1231

Washington
Washington State Psychiatric Association. 11626 13th Street S.W., Seattle WA 98146. (206) 248-3868

West Virginia
West Virginia Psychiatric Association. P.O. Box 630, West Virginia Medical Center, Department of Behavioral Medicine/Psychiatry, Morgantown WV 26506. (304) 293-2411

Wisconsin
Wisconsin Psychiatric Association. P.O. Box 1109, Madison WI 53701. (608) 257-6781

Wyoming
Wyoming Psychiatric Society. P.O. Box 1005, Cheyenne WY 82001. (307) 634-9653

Canada
Ontario District Branch of the American Psychiatric Association. 600 University Avenue, 9N, Room 942, Toronto, Ontario M5G 1X5. (416) 589-4569

Quebec & Eastern Canada District Branch of the American Psychiatric Association. Hospital Suite Therese, 1705 George Avenue, Shawinegan, Quebec G9N 2N1. (819) 537-9351

Western Canada District Branch of the American Psychiatric Association. Vancouver General Hospital, 715 West 12th Avenue, Vancouver, British Columbia V5Z 1M9. (604) 875-4515

American Psychological Association: Affiliated State Psychological Associations
Alabama Psychological Association. P.O. Box 97, Montgomery AL 36101-0097. (205) 262-8245

Alaska Psychological Association. Executive Officer, P.O. Box 230993, Anchorage AK 99523-0993. (907) 522-3802

Arizona Psychological Association. 202 E. McDowell Road, Suite 135, Phoenix AZ 85004-4533. (602) 253-3210

Arkansas Psychological Association. 3 Financial Center, 900 South Shackleford, Suite 300, Little Rock AR 72211. (501) 228-5550

California State Psychological Association. 1010 Eleventh Street, Suite 202, Sacramento CA 95814-3807. (916) 325-9786 (Referral service to psychologists available)

Colorado Psychological Association. 720 South Colorado Boulevard, Suite 465, Denver CO 80222-1915. (303) 692-9303 (Referral service to psychologists available)

Connecticut Psychological Association. 60 Washington Street, Suite 203, Hartford CT 06106. (203) 549-2445 (Referral service to psychologists available)

Delaware Psychological Association. P.O. Box 718, Claymont DE 19703. (302) 475-1574

District of Columbia Psychological Association. 1010 Hamlin Street N.E., Washington DC 20017. (202) 232-6713 (Referral service to psychologists available)

Florida Psychological Association. 408 Office Plaza, Tallahassee FL 32301-2757. (904) 656-2222

Georgia Psychological Association. 1800 Peachtree Street, N.W., Atlanta GA 30309. (404) 874-5219

Hawaii Psychological Association. P.O. Box 10465, Honolulu HI 96816. (808) 377-5992 (Referral service to psychologists available)

Idaho Psychological Association. 405 South 8th Street, Suite 365, Boise ID 83702-7100. (208) 345-3072

Illinois Psychological Association. 203 North Wabash, No. 1200, Chicago IL 60601-2413. (312) 372-7610

Indiana Psychological Association. 8335 Allison Pointe Trail, Suite 250, Indianapolis IN 46250. (317) 841-8038

Iowa Psychological Association. P.O. Box 320, Knoxville IA 50138-2212. (515) 828-5035

Kansas Psychological Association. 400 S.W. Croix, Topeka KS 66611-2251. (913) 267-7435

Kentucky Psychological Association. Keller Child Psychiatry Research Center, 120 Sears Avenue, Suite 202, Louisville KY 40207-5063. (502) 894-0777

Louisiana Psychological Association. P.O. Box 66924, Baton Rouge LA 70896-6924. (504) 344-8839

Maine Psychological Association. 12 Spruce Street, Box 5435, Augusta ME 04330. (207) 621-0732

Psychological Association of Manitoba. 1800-155 Carlton Street, Winnipeg, MB R3C 3HB. (204) 947-3698

Maryland Psychological Association. 1 Mall North, Suite 314, 10025 Governor Warfield Parkway, Columbia MD 21044. (410) 992-4258

Massachusetts Psychological Association. 14 Beacon Street, No. 704, Boston MA 02108. (617) 523-6320

Michigan Psychological Association. 18296 Middlebelt Road, Suite A, Livonia MI 48152-3614. (313) 525-0460

Minnesota Psychological Association. 1740 Rice Street, Suite 220, St. Paul MN 55113-6811. (612) 489-2964 (Referral service to psychologists available)

Mississippi Psychological Association. P.O. Box 1120, 812 North President Street, Jackson MS 39215. (601) 353-1672

Missouri Psychological Association. 101 East High Street, Jefferson City MO 65101-2989. (314) 634-8852

Montana Psychological Association. 324 Fuller Avenue, Helena MT 59601-5029. (406) 443-1570

Nebraska Psychological Association. 1044 H Street, Lincoln NE 68508-3169. (402) 475-0754 (Referral service to psychologists available)

Nevada Psychological Association. 432 Court Street, Suite 202, Reno NV 89501-1776. (702) 324-1194

New Hampshire Psychological Organization, Professional Services. 2½ Beacon Street, P.O. Box 1215, Concord NH 03301. (603) 225-9925

New Jersey Psychological Association. 349 East Northfield Road, Suite 211, Livingston NJ 07039-4806. (201) 535-9888 (Referral service to psychologists available)

New Mexico Psychological Association. 2425 San Pedro, N.E., Suite D, Albuquerque NM 87110. (505) 883-7376

New York State Psychological Association. 1529 Western Avenue, Albany NY 12203-3500. (518) 456-7735/9

North Carolina Psychological Association. 1004 Dresser Court, Suite 106, Raleigh NC 27609-7353. (919) 872-1005

North Dakota Psychological Association. North Central Human Services Center. 1249 South Highland Acres Road, Bismarck ND 58501-2486. (701) 223-9045

Ohio Psychological Association. 400 East Town Street, Suite 020, Columbus OH 43215-1599. (614) 224-0034 (Referral service to psychologists available)

Oklahoma Psychological Association. 708 N.E. 42nd Street, Oklahoma City OK 73105. (405) 424-0019

Oregon Psychological Association. 1750 S.W. Skyline Boulevard, Suite 224, Portland OR 97221-2545. (503) 292-4914

Pennsylvania Psychological Association. 416 Forster Street, Harrisburg PA 17102-1714. (717) 232-3817

Puerto Rico Psychological Association. P.O. Box 363435, San Juan PR 00936-3435. (809) 751-7100

Rhode Island Psychological Association. Independence Square, 500 Prospect Street, Pawtucket RI 02860. (401) 728-5570

South Carolina Psychological Association. P.O. Box 5207, Columbia SC 29250. (803) 771-6050 (Referral service to psychologists available)

South Dakota Psychological Association. 1249 South Highland Acres Road, Bismarck ND 58501-2486. (701) 223-3184

Tennessee Psychological Association. 530 Church Street, Suite 300, Nashville TN 37219-2394. (615) 254-3687

Texas Psychological Association. 6633 East Highway 290, Suite 305, Austin TX 78723-1158. (512) 454-2449

Utah Psychological Association. 2102 East 3780 South, Salt Lake City UT 84109. (801) 278-4016

Vermont Psychological Association. P.O. Box 1017, Montpelier VT 05602. (802) 229-5447

Virginia Psychological Association. 109 Amherst Street, Winchester VA 22601. (703) 667-5544

Washington State Psychological Association. 13500 Lake City Way Northeast, No. 208, Seattle WA 98125. (206) 363-9772. (Referral service to psychologists available)

West Virginia Psychological Association. P.O. Box 667, Charleston WV 25323. (304) 345-2716

Wisconsin Psychological Association. 121 South Hancock Street, Madison WI 53703. (608) 251-1450

Wyoming Psychological Association. P.O. Box 1191, Laramie WY 82070. (307) 745-3846

Canada

Ontario Psychological Association. 730 Yonge Street, Suite 221, Toronto, Ontario M4Y 2B7. (416) 961-5552 (Referral service to psychologists available)

Corporation Professionnelle des Psychologues du Quebec (CPPQ), 1100 Rue Beaumont, Ville Mont-Royal, Quebec H3P 3E5. (514) 738-1881 (Referral service to psychologists available)

National Association of Social Workers: Chapter Offices

Alabama Chapter, NASW. 2921 Marti Lane, Suite G, Montgomery AL 36116. (205) 288-2633

Alaska Chapter, NASW. 8923 Tanis Drive, Juneau AK 99801. (907) 789-7099

Arizona Chapter, NASW. 610 West Broadway, Suite 218, Tempe AZ 85281. (602) 968-4595

Arkansas Chapter, NASW. 1123 South University, Suite 1010, Little Rock AR 72204. (501) 663-0658

California Chapter, NASW. 1016 23rd Street, Sacramento CA 95816. (916) 442-4565

California Chapter, NASW. L. A. Branch Office, 6030 Wilshire Boulevard, Suite 202, Los Angeles CA 90036. (213) 935-2050

Colorado Chapter, NASW. 6000 East Evans, Building 1, Suite 121, Denver CO 80222. (303) 753-8890 or (303) 753-8891

Connecticut Chapter, NASW. 1800 Silas Deane Highway, Suite 20–21, Rocky Hill CT 06067. (203) 257-8066

Delaware Chapter, NASW. 3301 Green Street, Claymont DE 19703. (302) 792-0646

Metro Washington, District of Columbia, Chapter, NASW. 2025 Eye Street N. W., Suite 105, Washington DC 20006. (202) 457-0492

Florida Chapter, NASW. 345 South Magnolia Drive, No. 14B, Tallahassee FL 32301. (904) 224-2400 or (800) 352-6279

Georgia Chapter, NASW. 300 Wieuca Road, Suite 220, Atlanta GA 30342. (404) 255-6422

Hawaii Chapter, NASW. 245 North Kukui Street, Suite 206, Honolulu HI 96817. (808) 521-1787

Idaho Chapter, NASW. 200 North 4th Street, Boise ID 83702. (208) 343-2752

Illinois Chapter, NASW. 180 North Michigan Avenue, Suite 400, Chicago IL 60601. (312) 236-8308

Illinois Chapter, NASW, Springfield Branch Office. Lincoln Towers, 520 South 2nd Street, Suite 400, Springfield IL 60201. (217) 523-9303

Indiana Chapter, NASW. 1100 West 42nd Street, Suite 316, Indianapolis IN 46208. (317) 923-9878

International Chapter, NASW. CMR 419 Box, APO, AE 092, 011-49-622-131-5915

Iowa Chapter, NASW. 4211 Grand Avenue, Level 3, Des Moines IA 50312. (515) 277-1117

Kansas Chapter, NASW. Jayhawk Towers, 700 S.W. Jackson Street, Suite 901, Topeka KS 66603-3740. (913) 354-4804

Kentucky Chapter, NASW. 226 B West Second Street, P.O. Box 1211, Frankfort KY 40602. (502) 223-0245

Louisiana Chapter, NASW. LSU School of Social Work, 311 Huey Long Field House, Baton Rouge LA 70803. (504) 388-5437

Maine Chapter, NASW. 181 State Street, P.O. Box 5065, Augusta ME 04332. (207) 662-7592

Maryland Chapter, NASW. 5710 Executive Drive, Suite 105, Baltimore MD 21228. (301) 788-1066

Massachusetts Chapter, NASW. 14 Beacon Street, Suite 409, Boston MA 02108. (617) 227-9635

Michigan Chapter, NASW. 230 North Washington Square, Suite 212, Lansing MI 48933. (517) 487-1548

Minnesota Chapter, NASW. 480 Concordia Avenue, St. Paul MN 55103. (612) 293-1935

Mississippi Chapter, NASW. P.O. Box 4228, Jackson MS 39216. (601) 981-8359

Missouri Chapter, NASW. Parkade Center, Suite 138, 601 Business Loop 70 West, Columbia MO 65203. (314) 874-6140; (800) 333-6279

Montana Chapter, NASW. 555 Fuller Avenue, Helena MT 59715. (406) 499-6206

Nebraska Chapter, NASW. 1701 South 17th Street, Suite 1-E, Lincoln NE 68502. (402) 477-7344

Nevada Chapter, NASW. P.O. Box 50352, Henderson NV 89016. (702) 456-0046

New Hampshire Chapter, NASW. c/o New Hampshire Association for the Blind, 25 Walker Street, Concord NH 03301. (603) 224-4039

New Jersey Chapter, NASW. 110 West State Street, Trenton NJ 08608. (609) 394-1666

New Mexico Chapter, NASW. 1503 University Boulevard N.E., Albuquerque NM 87102. (505) 247-2336

New York City Chapter, NASW. 545 8th Avenue, 6th Floor, New York NY 10018. (212) 947-5000

New York State Chapter, NASW. 225 Lark Street, Albany NY 12210. (518) 463-4741; (800) 724-6279

North Carolina Chapter, NASW. P.O. Box 27582, Raleigh NC 27611-7582. (919) 828-9650

North Dakota Chapter, NASW. P.O. Box 1775, Jamestown ND 58502-1775. (701) 223-4161

Ohio Chapter, NASW. 42 East Gay Street, Suite 700, Columbus OH 43215. (614) 461-4484

Oklahoma Chapter, NASW. P.O. Box 2609, Norman OK 73070. (405) 329-7003

Oregon Chapter, NASW. 7688 S.W. Capital Highway, Portland OR 97219. (503) 452-8420

Pennsylvania Chapter, NASW. 1007 North Front Street, Suite 2 North, Harrisburg PA 17102. (717) 232-4125

Puerto Rico Chapter, NASW. D-3 Via Bernardo, Monte Alvernia, Guaynabo PR 00969. (809) 758-3588

Rhode Island Chapter, NASW. 1736 Post Road, Warwick RI 02888. (401) 732-4340

South Carolina Chapter, NASW. P.O. Box 5008, Columbia SC 29250. (803) 256-8406

South Dakota Chapter, NASW. 4961 Sheridan Lake Road, Rapid City SD 57702. (605) 341-0526

Tennessee Chapter, NASW. 1720 West End Avenue, Suite 504, Nashville TN 37204. (615) 321-5095

Texas Chapter, NASW. 810 West 11th Street, Austin TX 78701. (512) 474-1454 or (800) 888-6279

Utah Chapter, NASW. University of Utah Graduate School of Social Work, Salt Lake City UT 84112. (801) 583-8855

Vermont Chapter, NASW. P.O. Box 147, Woodstock VT 05091. (802) 457-3645

Virgin Islands Chapter, NASW. Havensight Secretarial Services, 2 Buccaneer Mall, St. Thomas, VI 00820. (809) 776-3424

Virginia Chapter, NASW. The Virginia Building, 1 North 5th Street, Suite 410, Richmond VA 23219. (804) 643-1833

Washington Chapter, NASW. 2366 Eastlake Avenue East, Suite 236, Seattle WA 98102. (206) 325-9791

West Virginia Chapter, NASW. 1608 Virginia Street East, Charleston WV 25311. (304) 343-6141

Wisconsin Chapter, NASW. 14 Mifflin Street, Suite 104, Madison WI 53703. (608) 257-6334

Wyoming Chapter, NASW. 3001 Henderson Drive, Suite I, Cheyenne WY 82001. (307) 634-7763

Europe
European Chapter, NASW. 147th Postal Unit, Box R-207, APO, NY 09102. 49-6221-37481

National Mental Health Association: Affiliated Divisions/Chapters

Alabama
Mental Health Association in Alabama. 306 Whitman Street, Montgomery AL 36104. (205) 834-3857

Alaska
Alaska Mental Health Association. 4050 Lake Otis Parkway, Suite 202, Anchorage, AK 99508. (907) 563-0880

Arizona
Arizona Mental Health Association. 3627 East Indian School, Suite 107, Phoenix AZ 85018. (602) 381-1591

Arkansas
Mental Health Association in Northwest Arkansas. P.O. Box 1993, Fayetteville AR 72702. (501) 521-1158

California
Mental Health Association in California. 926 J Street, Suite 611, Sacramento CA 95814. (916) 441-4627

Florida
Mental Health Association of Florida. 2337 Wednesday Street, Tallahassee FL 32308. (904) 385-7527

Georgia
Mental Health Association of Georgia. 1244 Clairmont Road, Suite 204, Decatur GA 30030. (404) 634-2850

Hawaii
Mental Health Association of Hawaii. 200 North Vineyard Boulevard, No. 507, Honolulu HI 96817. (808) 521-1846

Idaho
Mental Health Association in Idaho. 715 South Capitol Boulevard, Suite 401, Boise ID 83702. (208) 343-4866

Kentucky
Kentucky Mental Health Association. 400 Sherbum Lane, Suite 357, Louisville KY 40207. (502) 893-0460

Louisiana
Mental Health Association of Louisiana. 6700 Plaza Drive, Suite 104, New Orleans LA 70127. (504) 241-3462

Maryland
Mental Health Association of Maryland. 323 East 25th Street, 2nd Floor. Baltimore MD 21218. (301) 235-1178

Michigan
Mental Health Association in Michigan. 15920 West Twelve Mile Road, Southfield MI 48076. (313) 557-6777

Nebraska
Mental Health Association in Nebraska. 4600 Valley Road, Room 411, Lincoln NE 68510. (402) 488-1080

New Jersey
Mental Health Association in New Jersey. 60 South Fullerton Avenue, Room 105, Montclair NJ 07042. (201) 744-2500

New York
Mental Health Association in New York State. 75 New Scotland Avenue, Albany NY 12208. (518) 434-0439

North Carolina
Mental Health Association in North Carolina. 115½ West Morgan Street, Raleigh NC 27601. (919) 828-8145

Oklahoma
Mental Health Association in Oklahoma County. 5104 North Francis, Suite B (Shartel Shopping Center), Oklahoma City OK 73118. (405) 524-6363

Mental Health Association in Tulsa. 1502 South Denver, Tulsa OK 74119. (918) 585-1213

Rhode Island
Mental Health Association of Rhode Island. 855 Waterman Avenue, Suite D, East Providence RI 02914. (401) 431-1240

South Carolina
Mental Health Association in South Carolina. 1823 Gadsden Street, Columbia SC 29201. (803) 779-5363

Tennessee
Mental Health Association in Tennessee. 1844 Stonebrook Drive, Knoxville TN 37923. (615) 637-8210, 690-1175

Texas
Mental Health Association in Texas. 8401 Shoal Creek Boulevard, Austin TX 78758. (512) 454-3706

Utah
Mental Health Association in Utah. 255 East 400 South, Suite 150, Salt Lake City UT 84111. (801) 531-8996

Appendix D

RESOURCE ORGANIZATIONS FOR SPECIAL DISEASES AND PROBLEM AREAS

Alzheimer's Disease
Alzheimer's Association. 919 North Michigan Avenue, 10th floor, Chicago IL 60611. (800) 272-3900; (312) 335-8700

Amyotrophic Lateral Sclerosis (ALS)
ALS Association. 21021 Ventura Boulevard, Suite 321, Woodland Hills, CA 91364. (818) 340-7500

ALS Neuromuscular Research Foundation. 2351 Clay Street, Room 416, San Francisco CA 94115. (415) 923-3604

Brain Tumor
Acoustic Neuroma Association. P.O. Box 12402, Atlanta GA 30355. (404) 237-8023

American Brain Tumor Association (formerly Association for Brain Tumor Research). 3725 North Talman Avenue, Chicago IL 60618. (312) 286-5571; (800) 886-2282 (patient hotline)

American Cancer Society. 1599 Clifton Road N.E., Atlanta GA 30329. (404) 320-3333; (800) ACS-2345 (cancer information number)

Cancer Information Service. 1100 Glendon Avenue, Suite 711, Los Angeles CA 90024. (310) 206-0278; (800) 4-CANCER

National Brain Tumor Foundation. 323 Geary Street, No. 510, San Francisco CA 94102. (415) 296-0404

Other Brain Diseases/Disorders

Alliance of Genetic Support Groups. 35 Wisconsin Circle, Suite 440, Chevy Chase MD 20815. (301) 652-5553; (800) 336-GENE; (301) 654-0171 (FAX)

American Academy of Neurology. 2221 University Avenue S.E., No. 335, Minneapolis MN 55414. (612) 623-8115; (612) 623-3504 (FAX)

American Chronic Pain Association. P.O. Box 850, Rocklin CA 95677. (916) 632-0922; (916) 632-3208 (FAX)

American Lupus Society. 5410 Wilshire Boulevard, Suite 611, Los Angeles CA 90036. (213) 933-4667

Chronic Fatigue Immune Dysfunction Syndrome Society. P.O. Box 230108, Portland OR 97223. (800) 442-3437

Dystonia Medical Research Foundation. 8383 Wilshire Boulevard, Suite 800, Beverly Hills CA 90211. (213) 852-1630

Epilepsy Foundation of America. 4351 Garden City Drive, Landover MD 20785. (301) 459-3700; (800) 332-1000; (301) 577-9056 (FAX)

Guardians of Hydrocephalus Research Foundation. 2618 Avenue Z, Brooklyn NY 11235. (718) 743-4473; (800) 458-8655; (718) 743-1171 (FAX)

Guillian-Barre Syndrome Foundation Support Group International. P.O. Box 262, Wynnewood PA 19096. (215) 667-0131

Lupus Foundation of America. 4 Research Place, Suite 180, Rockville MD 20850-3226. (301) 670-9292; (800) 558-0121 (recording); (301) 670-9486 (FAX)

Lupus Foundation of America, Southern California Chapter. 14600 (Golden West, No. 105–106, Westminster CA 92683. (714) 891-6400; (800) 426-6026 (in CA)

Malignant Hyperthermia Association of the United States. P.O. Box 191, Westport CT 06881-0191. (203) 655-3007

Muscular Dystrophy. 3561 East Sunrise Drive, Tucson AZ 85718. (602) 529-2000; (602) 529-5300 (FAX)

National AIDS Information Clearinghouse. P.O. Box 6003, Rockville MD 20850. (800) 458-5231

National Ataxia Foundation. 750 Twelve Oaks Center, 15500 Wayzata Boulevard, Wayzata MN 55391. (612) 473-7666; (612) 473-9289 (FAX)

National Center for the Study of Wilson's Disease. Albert Einstein College of Medicine, 1300 Morris Park Avenue, Bronx NY 10461. (212) 892-5119; (212) 863-7572 (FAX)

National Epilepsy Library. 4351 Garden City Drive, Landover MD 20785. (301) 459-3700; (800) 332-4050; (301) 577-2684 (FAX)

National Foundation for Brain Research. 1250 24th Street N.W., Suite 600, Washington DC 20037. (202) 293-5453; (202) 466-2888 (FAX)

National Headache Foundation (formerly National Migraine Foundation). 5252 North Western Avenue, Chicago IL 60625. (312) 878-7715

National Hydrocephalus Foundation. 400 North Michigan, Suite 1102, Chicago IL 60611-4102. (815) 467-6548

National Institute of Neurological Disorders and Stroke. Building 31, Room 8A-06, Bethesda MD 20892. (301) 496-5751; (800) 352-9424 (recording); (301) 402-2186 (FAX)

National Multiple Sclerosis Society. 733 Third Avenue, 6th Floor, New York NY 10017. (212) 986-3240; (800) 227-3166; (212) 986-7981 (FAX)

National Neurofibromatosis Foundation. 141 Fifth Avenue, Suite 7S, New York NY 10010. (212) 460-8980; (800) 323-7938

National Organization for Rare Disorders. P.O. Box 8923, New Fairfield CT 06812. (203) 746-6518; (800) 999-6673; (203) 746-6481 (FAX)

National Society of Genetic Counselors. 2333 Canterbury Drive, Waulingford PA 19086. (written inquiries only)

National Tuberous Sclerosis Association, Inc. 8000 Corporate Drive, Suite 120, Landover MD 20785. (301) 459-9888; (800) 225-NTSA; (301) 459-0394 (FAX)

Parent Council for Growth Normality (Creutzfeldt-Jakob Disease). 664 South Market Street, Opelousas LA 70570. (318) 942-9700

Society for Progressive Supra Nuclear Palsy. c/o David Saks, 2904-B Marnat Road, Baltimore MD 21209. (301) 484-8771

Tourettes Syndrome Association, Inc., 42-40 Bell Boulevard, Bayside NY 11361. (718) 224-2999; (800) 237-0717; (718) 279-9596 (FAX)

United Cerebral Palsy Association, Inc. 7 Penn Plaza, Suite 804, New York NY 10001. (212) 520-1776

Vestibular Disorders Association. P.O. Box 4467, Portland OR 97208-4467. (503) 279-7705; (503) 229-8064 (FAX)

Wilson's Disease Association. P.O. Box 75324, Washington DC 20013. (703) 636-3003; (703) 636-3014

Caregivers/Family
Children of Aging Parents. Woodburn Office Campus, 1609 Woodburn Road, Suite 302A, Levittown PA 19057. (215) 945-6900

Elder Care America, Inc. 1141 Loxford Terrace, Silver Spring MD 20901. (301) 593-1621

Family Service America. 11700 West Lake Park Drive, Milwaukee WI 53224. (414) 359-1040

Family Survival Project. 425 Bush Street, Suite 500, San Francisco CA 94108. (415) 434-3388; (800) 445-8106

National Federation of Interfaith Volunteer Caregivers, Inc. 105 Mary's Avenue, P.O. Box 1939, Kingston NY 12401. (914) 331-1358

Well Spouse Foundation. P.O. Box 28876, San Diego CA 92198-0876. (619) 673-9043; (914) 357-8513 (East Coast contact)

Death and Dying
Choice in Dying (Concern for Dying Educational Counsel). 200 Varick Street, New York NY 10014. (212) 366-5540

Compassionate Friends, Inc. P.O. Box 3696, Oakbrook IL 60522-3696. (708) 990-0010

Foundation for Hospice and Homecare. 519 C Street N.E., Stanton Park, Washington DC 20002-5809. (202) 547-6586

National Hospice Organization. 1901 North Moore Street, Suite 901, Arlington VA 22209. (703) 243-5900

National Neurological Research Bank (Autopsies). V.A. Wadsworth Medical Center, Wilshire and Sawtelle Boulevards, Los Angeles CA 90073. (310) 824-4307

National Research and Information Center (Death, Grief and Funerals). 2250 East Devon Avenue, Suite 250, Des Plaines IL 60018. (800) 662-7666

Disability Associations
ABLEDATA (National Information Resource Center on Disability). c/o Springfield Center of Independent Living, 426 West Jefferson, Springfield IL 62702. (217) 523-2587

American Foundation for the Blind. 15 West 16th Street, New York NY 10011. (212) 620-2000

American Paralysis Association. 500 Morris Avenue, Springfield NJ 07081. (800) 225-0292 *or:* 2149 Seville Avenue, Balboa CA 92661. (714) 673-8474; (800) 527-5206

American Speech, Language, Hearing Association. 10801 Rockville Pike, Rockville MD 20852. (301) 897-8682 (Voice/TDD); (301) 571-0457 (FAX)

Association for Persons in Supported Employment. 5001 West Broad Street, Suite 34, Richmond VA 23230. (804) 282-3655

Help for Incontinent People. P.O. Box 544, Union SC 29379. (803) 579-7900

International Center for the Disabled. 340 East 24th Street, New York NY 10010. (212) 679-0100; (212) 889-0372 (TTY)

National Association for the Deaf. 814 Thayer Avenue, Silver Spring MD 20910. (301) 587-6282

National Center for Disability Services (formerly Human Resources Center). 201 I.U. Willets Road, Albertson NY 11507. (516) 747-5400; (516) 746-3298 (FAX)

National Council for Independent Living. 2111 Wilson Boulevard, Suite 405, Arlington VA 22201. (703) 525-3409; (703) 525-3409; (FAX) (703) 525-3407 (TTYD)

National Council on Disability. 800 Independence Avenue S.W., Suite 814, Washington DC 20591. (202) 267-3846; (202) 267-3232 (TDD)

National Easter Seal Society. 70 East Lake Street, Chicago IL 60601. (312) 726-6200

National Information Center for Children and Youths with Handicaps. P.O. Box 1492, Washington DC 20013. (703) 893-6061; (800) 999-5599; (703) 893-1741 (FAX)

National Institute on Disability and Rehabilitation Research. 400 Maryland Avenue S.W., Washington, DC 20202-2572. (202) 732-1134

National Organization on Disability. 910 16th Street N.W., Suite 600, Washington DC 20006. (202) 293-5960

National Spinal Cord Injury Association. 600 West Cumming Park, Suite 2000, Woburn MA 01801. (617) 935-2722; (800) 962-9629 (Hotline)

Spinal Cord Society. Wendell Road, Fergus Falls MN 56537. (218) 739-5252; (218) 739-5262 (FAX)

World Institute on Disability. 510 16th Street, Suite 100, Oakland CA 94612-1502. (510) 763-4100; (510) 763-4109 (FAX)

Facilities/Placement
American Association of Homes for the Aging. 901 East Street N.W., Suite 500, Washington DC 20004. (202) 783-2242; (202) 783-2255 (FAX)

Commission on the Accreditation of Rehabilitation Facilities. 101 North Wilmot Road, No. 500, Tucson AZ 85711. (602) 748-1212; (602) 571-1601 (FAX)

Hillhaven Foundation. 1148 Broadway Plaza, Tacoma WA 99401-2264. (206) 572-4901

National Association of Rehabilitation Facilities. Post Office Drawer 17675. Washington DC 20041. (703) 648-9300; (800) 368-3513; (703) 648-0346 (FAX)

National Citizens Coalition for Nursing Home Reform. 1224 M Street N.W., Suite 301, Washington DC 20005. (202) 393-2018; (202) 393-4122 (FAX)

Shared Housing Resource Center. 6344 Greene Street, Philadelphia PA 19144. (215) 848-1220; (800) 677-7472

Head Trauma
Advocates for Highway and Auto Safety. 777 North Capitol Street N.E., Suite 410, Washington DC 20002. (202) 408-1711; (202) 408-1699 (FAX)

Brain Trauma Foundation. 555 Madison Avenue, Suite 2001, New York NY 10022-3303. (212) 753-5003; (212) 753-0149 (FAX)

Brown Schools, National Information and Referral Service. P.O. Box 4008, Austin TX 78765. (512) 329-8821; (800) 531-5305; (512) 314-5254 (FAX)

National Head Injury Foundation. 1140 Connecticut Avenue N.W., Washington DC 20036. (202) 296-6443; (800) 444-NHIF

Rehabilitation Research and Training Center, Community Integration of Persons with TBI. 194 Farber Hall, 3435 Main Street, Buffalo NY 14214. (716) 829-2300; (716) 829-2390 (FAX)

Rehabilitation Research and Training Center for Brain Injury and Stroke/Rehabilitation Medicine. University of Washington, Medicine RJ-30, Seattle WA 98195. (206) 543-3600; (206) 685-3244 (FAX)

Research and Training Center on Head Trauma and Stroke. 400 East 34th Street, New York NY 10016. (212) 263-6185

Home Care/Day Care
American Hospital Association (Ambulatory and Home Care Services). 840 North Lake Shore Drive, Chicago IL 60611. (312) 280-6000

National Association for Home Care. 519 C Street N.E., Stanton Park, Washington DC 20002. (202) 547-7424; (202) 547-3540

National Association of Private Geriatric Care Managers. 655 North Alvernon Way, Alvernon Place, Suite 108, Tucson AZ 85711. (602) 881-8008; (602) 325-7925 (FAX)

National Council of Senior Citizens, National Senior Citizens Education and Research, Inc. 1331 F Street N.W., Washington DC 20004. (202) 347-8800; (202) 624-9595 (FAX)

National Institute on Adult Day Care. c/o National Council on the Aging, 1409 3rd Street S.W., Suite 200, Washington DC 20024. (202) 479-1200; (800) 424-9046; (202) 479-0735 (FAX)

Visiting Nurses Association of America. 3801 East Florida Avenue, Suite 900, Denver CO 80210. (303) 753-0218; (800) 426-2547; (303) 753-0258 (FAX)

Huntington's Disease
Hereditary Disease Foundation. 1427 Seventh Street, Suite 2, Santa Monica CA 90401. (310) 458-4183; (310) 458-3937 (FAX)

Huntington's Disease Society of America, Inc. 140 West 22nd Street, Sixth Floor, New York NY 10011. (212) 242-1968; (800) 345-HDSA; (212) 243-2443 (FAX)

Legal Assistance
American Bar Association, Commission on Legal Problems of the Elderly. 1800 M Street N.W., Washington DC 20036. (202) 331-2297; (202) 331-2220 (FAX)

Legal Research and Services for the Elderly. 1331 F Street N.W., Washington DC 20004. (202) 347-8800; (202) 624-9595 (FAX)

National Academy of Elder Law Attorneys. 655 North Alvernon Way, Suite 108, Tucson AZ 85711. (602) 881-4005; (602) 325-7925 (FAX)

National Association of Protection and Advocacy Systems. 900 Second Street N.E., Suite 211, Washington DC 20002. (202) 408-9514; (202) 962-4210 (FAX)

National Clearinghouse for Legal Services. 407 South Dearborn Street, Suite 400, Chicago IL 60605. (312) 939-3830; (800) 621-3256; (312) 939-4536 (FAX)

National Employment Law Institute. 444 Magnolia Avenue, Suite 200, Larkspur CA 94939. (415) 924-3844; (415) 924-2908 (FAX)

National Health Law Program. 2639 South La Cienega Boulevard, Los Angeles CA 90034. (310) 204-6010; (310) 204-6891 (FAX)

National Health Lawyers Association. 1620 I Street N.W., Suite 900, Washington DC 20006. (202) 833-1100; (202) 833-1105 (FAX)

National Organization of Social Security Claimants Representatives. 6 Prospect Street, Midland Park NJ 07432. (201) 444-1415; (800) 431-2804; (201) 444-1823 (FAX)

National Senior Citizens Law Center. 1816 H Street N.W., Suite 700, Washington DC 20006. (202) 887-5280; (202) 785-6792 (FAX) *or:* 1052 West 6th Street, Suite 700, Los Angeles CA 90017. (213) 482-3550

Pension Rights Center. 918 16th Street, Suite 704, Washington DC 20006. (202) 296-3778; (202) 833-2472 (FAX)

Long-Term Care Policy
Families USA Foundation. 1334 G Street N.W., Washington DC 20005. (202) 628-3030; (202) 347-2417 (FAX)

Long Term Care Campaign. 1334 G Street N.W., Suite 500, Washington DC 20005. (202) 393-2092; (202) 393-2109 (FAX)

National Academy for State Health Policy. 50 Monument Square, Portland ME 04101. (207) 780-4948; (207) 874-6527 (FAX)

National Center for Social Policy and Practice. 750 First Street N.E., Washington DC 20002. (202) 495-7244; (800) 638-8799; (202) 336-8311 (FAX)

Robert Wood Johnson Foundation. Rt. 1 North and College Road East, P.O. Box 2316, Princeton NJ 08543-2316. (609) 452-8701

Washington Business Group on Health. 777 North Capitol Street N.E., Suite 800, Washington DC 20002. (202) 408-9320; (202) 408-9332

Parkinson's Disease
American Parkinson Disease Association, Inc. 60 Bay Street, Staten Island NY 10301. (718) 981-8001; (800) 223-APDA

American Parkinson Disease Association, Inc. West Coast National Office, 14551 Friar Street, Van Nuys CA 91411. (818) 908-9951; (818) 908-4331 (FAX)

National Parkinson Foundation. 1501 Northwest 9th Avenue, Bob Hope Road, Miami FL 33136. (305) 547-6666; (800) 327-4545; (305) 548-4403 (FAX)

National Parkinson Foundation. West Coast Office, 9911 West Pico Boulevard, Suite 500, Los Angeles CA 90035. (800) 400-8448 (in CA only); (800) 522-8855 (outside CA); (310) 203-8448; (310) 203-8459 (FAX)

Parkinson's Disease Foundation. William Black Medical Building, 640 West 168th Street, New York NY 10032. (212) 923-4700; (800) 457-6676; (212) 923-4770 (FAX)

Parkinson's Educational Program. 3900 Birch, Suite 105, Newport Beach, CA 92660. (714) 640-0218; (800) 344-7872; (714) 250-8530 (FAX)

Parkinson's Support Groups of America. 11376 Cherry Hill Road, Apt. 204, Beltsville MD 20705. (301) 937-1545

United Parkinson's Foundation. 360 West Superior Street, Chicago IL 60610. (312) 664-2344

Pharmacology
National Information Center for Orphan Drugs and Rare Diseases.
P.O. Box 1133, Washington DC 20013-1133. (800) 456-3505

Pharmaceutical Manufacturers Association Commission on Drugs for
Rare Diseases. 1100 15th Street N.W., Washington DC 20005. (202)
835-3560; (202) 785-4834 (FAX)

Rehabilitation
American Academy of Physical Medicine and Rehabilitation. 122 South
Michigan Avenue, Suite 1300, Chicago IL 60603-6107. (312) 922-9366;
(312) 922-6754 (FAX)

American Occupational Therapy Association. 1383 Piccard Drive,
P.O. Box 1725, Rockville MD 20849-1725. (301) 948-9626; (301)
948-5512 (FAX)

American Physical Therapy Association. 1111 North Fairfax Street, Alexandria VA 22314. (703) 684-2782

Brain Train. 727 Twinridge Lane, Richmond VA 23235. (804)
320-0105; (804) 320-0242 (FAX)

Council of State Administrators of Vocational Rehabilitation. P.O. Box
3776, Washington DC 20007. (202) 638-4634

National Rehabilitation Association. 1910 Association Drive, Suite 205,
Reston VA 22091. (703) 715-9090; (703) 715-1058 (FAX)

National Rehabilitation Information Center. 8455 Colesville Road, Suite
935, Silver Spring MD 20910-3319. (301) 588-9284; (800) 346-2742;
(301) 587-1967 (FAX)

Research and Training Center on Independent Living at TM. 2323
South Shepherd, Suite 1000, Houston TX 77019. (713) 520-0732;
(713) 520-5136 (TDD); (713) 520-5785 (FAX)

Upledger Institute (Craniosacral Therapy). 11211 Prosperity Farms
Road, Palm Beach Gardens FL 33410. (407) 622-4334; (407) 622-4771
(FAX)

Stroke
American Heart Association, National Center (Stroke Clubs). 7272
Greenville Avenue, Dallas TX 75231. (214) 373-6300; (214) 706-1341
(FAX)

Courage Stroke Network. 3915 Golden Valley Road, Golden Valley MN 55422. (800) 553-6321; (612) 520-0577 (FAX)

National Stroke Association. 300 East Hampton Avenue, Suite 240, Englewood CO 80110-2654. (303) 762-9922; (800) 787-6537; (303) 762-1190 (FAX)

Stroke Club International. 805 12th Street, Galveston TX 77550. (409) 762-1022

INDEX

managing emotions and finding,
88–90
self-help groups, 30
Helplessness, feelings of, 67
Holmes, Thomas, 172
Homemakers, 223–24
Homes/housing
importance of, 19
in-home health aid, 223
nursing homes as, 20, 183–84,
190–91, 215–16
repair services, 224
sources of information on, 214–16,
256, 257
use of supportive, 183–84, 190–91
Horowitz, Mardi, 50
Huntington's disease, sources of
information on, 257–58

Idaho
Mental Health Association, 249
National Association of Social
Workers, 246
psychiatric society, 236
psychological society, 242
state agency on aging, 228
Illinois
National Association of Social
Workers, 246
psychiatric society, 236
psychological society, 242
state agency on aging, 228
Indiana
National Association of Social
Workers, 246
psychiatric societies, 236
psychological society, 242
state agency on aging, 228
Inferences about the unknown, 75
Information
denial and processing, 51
emotional states and seeking, 75
investigating and obtaining,
125–26
Iowa
National Association of Social
Workers, 246
psychiatric society, 236

psychological society, 242
state agency on aging, 228

Kansas
National Association of Social
Workers, 246
psychiatric society, 237
psychological society, 242
state agency on aging, 228
Kentucky
Mental Health Association, 249
National Association of Social
Workers, 246
psychiatric society, 237
psychological society, 242
state agency on aging, 228
Keyes, Ralph, 181

Labeling, 74–75
Leadership, alternate, in family, 139
Legal documents, 186, 193–94
Legal matters, sources of information
on, 217, 258
Letting go, 17–19
of belief one directs one's parents'
lives, 182, 185–87
establishing emotional distance, 183,
189–90
letting others help, 182, 188–89
moving on, 184, 204–8
phases, 181–82
preparing for death, 184, 191–204
setting limits, 182, 187–88
use of supportive housing/nursing
home, 183–84, 190–91
Limits
setting, 182, 187–88
understanding, 21–22
Listening, active, 142
Lithium carbonate, 92
Living wills, 186, 193
Long-term care policy, sources of
information on, 258–59
Louisiana
Mental Health Association, 249
National Association of Social
Workers, 246
psychiatric society, 237

The "intellectual & cognitive chang of advanced aging..."